Naturally Healthy with

Evening Primrose Oil

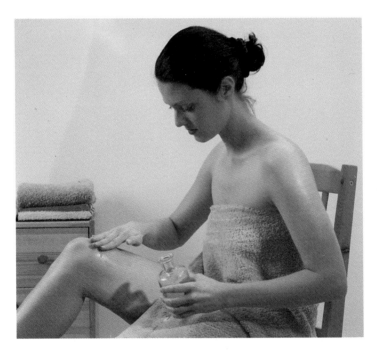

Werner Meidinger

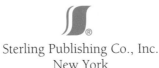

Sterling Publishing Co., Inc.
New York

**Library of Congress
Cataloging-in-Publication
Data Available**

10 9 8 7 6 5 4 3 2 1

Published by Sterling
    Publishing Company, Inc.
    387 Park Avenue South,
    New York, N.Y. 10016
Originally published in
    Germany under the title
    *Natürlich gesund mit
    Nachtkerzenöl* and © 1998
    by W. Ludwig Buch verlag,
    a part of Sudwest Verlag
    GmbH & Co. KG,
    München
Translation © 1999 by Sterling
    Publishing Company, Inc.
Distributed in Canada by
    Sterling Publishing
    c/o Canadian Manda Group,
    One Atlantic Avenue, Suite
    105, Toronto, Ontario,
    Canada M6K 3E7
Distributed in Great Britain
    and Europe by Cassell PLC
    Wellington House, 125
    Strand, London
    WC2R 0BB, England
Distributed in Australia by
    Capricorn Link (Australia)
    Pty Ltd. P.O. Box 6651,
    Baulkham Hills, Business
    Centre, NSW 2153,
    Australia
*Manufactured in the United
    States of America*
All rights reserved

Sterling ISBN 0-8069-2035-1

Contents

Evening primrose flowers are a vibrant yellow color.

Preface

Approximately 500 years ago, various North American indigenous tribes coveted the common evening primrose (*Oenothera biennis*) plant for its valuable healing and nutritive properties. They used its tender leaves and strong roots as a vegetable. The tips of the stalks and other parts of the plant that they removed during its first year of growth were stored in oil and served cold as an accompaniment to different foods.

An Herb for Nourishment and Healing

In addition to being valued as a vegetable, evening primrose was highly sought after for the treatment of various ailments. A syrup prepared from its flowers was used in alleviating symptoms of asthma and whooping cough and for digestive problems and disorders of the gastrointestinal tract. The medicine men of the Iroquois tribe prepared medications from evening primrose in order to heal running sores and to strengthen their muscles. The Cherokees used its leaves in a tea to cure diarrhea and as an aid in weight reduction. The Navajos used various parts of the plant for medicinal purposes either ground up into a fine meal or as a tea or a syrup. They also cooked its roots and stalks, and ate them as vegetables. In its various forms of application, evening primrose was utilized for the treatment of colds, rheumatic disorders, and stomach and digestive problems. The plant was even used to help cure female disorders and heal ulcers.

The Discovery of Evening Primrose Oil

The first references to the healing properties of the oil from the evening primrose plant are found among the Algonquins. They mashed its oily seeds and applied this paste as a poultice for skin rashes. Algonquin women also used this remedy for cosmetic purposes. Regular applications of the paste prepared from evening primrose were thought to guarantee smooth and youthful skin.

The evening primrose plant has roots up to 2 inches (5 centimeters) thick and 4 inches (10 centimeters) long. The Navajo Indians used to dig up these roots in the fall and grind them into a fine powder. This powder was then mixed with water or milk and used as a compress for hemorrhoids.

The Rediscovery of a Traditional Healing Plant

Apart from the indigenous tribes just mentioned and a few European settlers in North America who appear to have made use of the evening primrose plant, it seems that everyone else had forgotten its manifold healing properties. It was only in 1749 that Peter Kalm, a Swedish botanist, rediscovered evening primrose as a natural healing remedy. Following this, studies were made of old herbal reference books and tests were conducted on patients. These tests showed such overwhelming success that in 1868 evening primrose was placed on Canada's official list of healing plants. Over the last ten decades, scientists all over the world have studied the healing applications of evening primrose and other herbs, bringing about a renaissance in the area of phytotherapy (the use of vegetable drugs in medicine).

This book describes some of the latest findings regarding the active ingredients of evening primrose, as it is used in the areas of medicine and cosmetics, and gives you many tips for the herb's practical application. We have also included some recipes that are simple to use on a daily basis, in order to improve your mental and physical well-being in a totally natural way through the use of the plant's oil, leaves, tips, and roots.

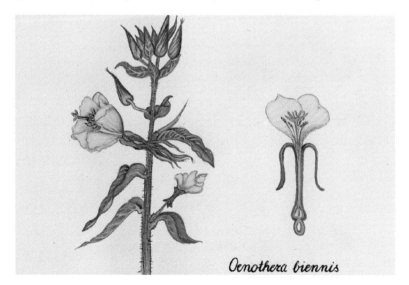

Oenothera biennis

"The leaves and roots of evening primrose were used as a blood-purifying remedy. In naturopathy, preparations from evening primrose have long been used successfully against diarrhea. In more recent times, the oil from evening primrose has been shown to be especially effective in the treatment of various illnesses."
—Dr. Helmut Pabst, Education Chairman of the Bavarian Association for Sports Medicine

Oenothera biennis means biennial evening primrose.

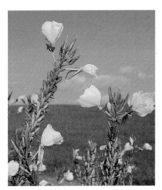

Evening primrose blooms at night and has a vertical growth pattern, reminding one of a candle.

The blossoms of evening primrose have a bright yellow glow. They are about an inch (2 to 3 centimeters) long and up to 2.5 inches (45 millimeters) wide. The calyx is surrounded by four heart-shaped crown petals. The eight stamens are arranged in two circles.

A Brief Lesson in Botany

A Healing Remedy with a Long Tradition

Originally, the evening primrose plant grew only in North America. It was not until the early seventeenth century that its seeds reached Europe. In 1612, evening primrose was cultivated as a decorative plant in the Botanical Garden of Padua in northeastern Italy. From there, it spread as a wildflower all over Europe. Evening primrose is also known as tree primrose, German rampion, scabbish, scurvish, sundrop, kings' cure-all, and nightwillow herb.

Other varieties from the nightshade plant family had been known in Europe long before the spread of evening primrose. Its generic name *Oenothera* can be traced back as far as antiquity, when it was established by Theophrastus (372–287 B.C.), a student of Aristotle. The ancient Greeks enjoyed snacking on the roots of the then-known nightshade plants while drinking wine. *Oenothera* is derived from the Greek word *oinos,* which means wine. Legend has it that evening primrose plants sprinkled with wine were supposedly capable of taming wild animals. This may explain the second part of its name: *thera,* which refers to a wild animal or a hunt.

From Antiquity to Modern Times

Today, the common evening primrose (*Oenothera biennis*) can be found throughout Europe. It grows along trails, railroad embankments, by the side of the road, in waste piles, or in stone quarries—in short, wherever there is poor and sandy soil.

Some Botanical Data

During its first year, the biennial plant (*biennis*) will grow nothing more than a leafy rosette close to the ground. It is only in its second season that the plant develops its flowering stalk, which grows to more than 3 feet (1 meter) high. Its vibrant yellow flowers will bloom from June through October. The blossoms are pollinated predominantly by nocturnal butterflies, which are attracted by their fragrance. Until the fall, each blossom will bear a seed capsule containing approximately 200 seeds, which are up to ⅛ of an inch (2 millimeters) long. Approximately 5,000 seed capsules are needed in order to obtain a mere 500 milligrams of evening primrose oil.

Extracting the Oil

There are various processes for the extraction of traditional vegetable oils from the fruit and the seeds of different plants. The most commonly used procedures include mechanical pressing, extraction through chemicals, and centrifugal processing. During mechanical pressing, wedge presses squeeze the oil from the seeds or the fruit. In the production of industrially processed oils, the pressure and the preheating of the fruit or the seed mass result in relatively high temperatures (the oil yield rises with increasing temperature), but valuable ingredients are sometimes destroyed in the process.

During a cold pressing, which eliminates the preheating stage, temperatures may still reach 162°F (70°C), which is capable of damaging the valuable oils from the evening primrose plant if not destroying them altogether. This is why a special Cryo-Press cold procedure was developed to extract the oil from the evening primrose plant. Carbon dioxide, a natural substance that is not dangerous to our health, is applied to the seed capsules under high pressure and extracts the oil without generating any significant temperature levels.

In earlier times, the stalks and the leaves of the evening primrose plant were used mainly for a topical treatment in the healing of wounds, because they contain a number of ingredients that are capable of reducing skin inflammations as well as fighting the danger of fungal infections and certain types of viruses or bacteria. Today, it is mostly the oil pressed from the seeds that is used externally as well as internally for a variety of afflictions, including cardiovascular problems, neurodermatitis, and gynecological disorders.

The Flower of the Night

The plant itself is as captivating as its multifaceted healing powers. As its name implies, its blossoms open up only at night. It is not until six or seven o'clock in the evening that evening primrose unfolds its full beauty. Just before sunrise, the blossoms will close up again. But this color display will last for only a very short duration. From the time that a blossom first opens, it will be a mere twenty-four hours until it will already begin to wilt!

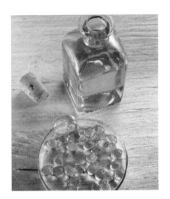

Evening primrose oil is available in liquid form or in capsules.

The oil from the evening primrose plant doesn't look any different from that from other plants. It is a yellowish color, and its aroma is reminiscent of poppy seed oil. However, due to its high content of essential fatty acids, evening primrose oil is qualitatively a much more valuable oil than other types of vegetable oil.

Ready-Made Products or Homegrown?

Ready-to-Use Oil

Pure evening primrose oil can be purchased at pharmacies and health food stores or by ordering it through the mail. For the best results, you should always make sure that you are buying a high-quality cold-pressed oil.

Administration and Application

There are various brands of evening primrose oil offered in capsule form. As a rule, each capsule contains 500 mg of oil. In the United States, the price for sixty 500 mg capsules is about $6. You should follow the manufacturer's recommendations as to dosage. A 2-ounce bottle of the oil runs about $18 in the United States. The applications described in this book require only a few drops in each instance, so this amount will last for a considerable length of time. Although evening primrose oil may appear more expensive than other oils initially, it compares favorably on a long-term basis due to its high content of natural healing components.

Homegrown Evening Primrose

If you have your own garden, you can cultivate the plant yourself. In earlier times, a typical farmer's garden would often feature evening primrose as a favorite and popular vegetable plant. It makes no demands on the soil and requires little care. And you can prepare herbal teas as well as healthful dishes from its stalks, leaves, and roots.

Cultivation: An Easy Process

Evening primrose seeds can be purchased at special nurseries. But you can also simply gather the seeds yourself in the fall from plants growing in the wild.

In places where there is a harsh climate in the winter, the best time for planting is the spring, from roughly April onward, when there is no more danger of frost. The seeds should be planted in boxes in a protected location. The germination rate is relatively high. Approximately 70 percent of the seeds show their first tender shoots within fifteen to thirty days. You can then transplant the seedlings into open beds from May onward.

Harvesting Evening Primrose

Evening primrose is a biennial plant, so you can harvest it only in its second year after starting it from seed. It is therefore recommended to alternate new crops every other year in two separate beds; this way, one generation will ripen annually and you don't have to wait until the following year to enjoy the fresh stalks, leaves, and roots.

If the leaves and the tips of the stalks are picked sparingly so that only a good third of the plant is harvested, it will continue to grow into the fall. You can then gather new seeds for the planting next spring and harvest enough roots for the preparation of vegetables and salads.

Recipes with which you can promote your health by preventing and treating certain illnesses are found in the chapter "Cooking with Evening Primrose Oil," starting on page 82.

Vitamin E is frequently added to evening primrose oil. This vitamin acts as an antioxidant, which means that it will protect the valuable unsaturated fatty acids from oxidation, or reaction with oxygen. Some manufacturers increase the durability of the vital unsaturated fatty acids in evening primrose oil through the addition of vitamin E.

Storing Evening Primrose Oil

Under normal circumstances, evening primrose oil can be stored without any problems for up to two years after opening. However, the unsaturated fatty acids contained in it tend to oxidize easily at room temperature, which results in a rancid odor and taste. In order to avoid this process, evening primrose oil should always be stored in the refrigerator.

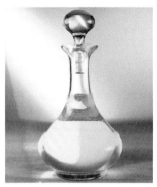

The valuable ingredients in evening primrose oil are its special essential fatty acids.

The Active Ingredients of Evening Primrose Oil

Fatty Acids

Each seed of the evening primrose plant consists of 24 percent proteins and 15 percent oil, apart from a wide range of other elements. It is this oil, in particular, that is so essential to our health, as it contains 71 percent linoleic acid and between 8 and 10 percent gamma-linolenic acid.

What Are Essential Fatty Acids?

Linoleic acid and gamma-linolenic acid are essential fatty acids. A substance is called "essential" when it is vital to the body's functioning but cannot be produced by the body itself, so it has to be ingested in sufficient amounts through the intake of food, for example.

Deficiency in Essential Fatty Acids

There are only a few plants that produce the valuable gamma-linolenic acid. In addition to evening primrose, they include borage, black currant, hemp, and black caraway.

In animal studies, a deficiency in essential fatty acids has shown to result in extremely deteriorated states of health. These health impairments range from retarded growth and a strongly diminished capacity in the healing of wounds to hair loss, pathologically enlarged oil glands, and skin eczema all the way to a progressive malfunctioning of the kidneys with subsequent kidney failure. Diminished liver activity, internal bleeding, a lack of tear and saliva fluid, and even infertility are the consequences. What follow are two descriptions in medical literature dealing with the effects of an essential fatty acids deficiency in the human body:

❦ During the fifties, an artificially produced breast-milk substitute became available for the first time for mothers who were unable or unwilling to nurse their babies. Because not much was known about essential fatty acids at that time, and especially not about their daily minimum requirement, too little of them was added to these milk preparations. The consequences: Babies who received the artificial breast-milk substitute suffered relatively soon after from eczema-like skin rashes. Those who did not have a severe reaction still suffered within a relatively short period of time from overly dry and scaly skin. When the proportion of essential fatty acids was increased later on, these skin rashes disappeared.

❦ During the seventies, the FDA in the United States prohibited the enrichment of intravenous food with essential fatty acids for patients who had to be fed intravenously in hospitals. Following this FDA ruling, adults as well were soon exhibiting eczemalike skin rashes, psoriasis, painful skin irritations, and a prolonged healing of wounds. Immediately after the FDA ban was lifted, the number of patients who had been fed intravenously and subsequently suffered from these skin disorders decreased dramatically.

Not only irritated skin but also healthy dry skin can profit from the active ingredients in evening primrose oil. The essential fatty acids that it contains support the natural functions of the skin and prevent its premature aging.

Comparison of Vegetable Oils

Vegetable Oils (Average Values)	Linoleic Acid	Gamma-Linolenic Acid
Evening primrose oil	71 %	9 %
Sunflower oil	60 %	–
Hemp seed oil	57 %	2 %
Corn oil	55 %	–
Peanut oil	26 %	–
Linseed oil	15 %	–
Olive oil	6 %	–
Borage oil	–	24 %
Currant seed oil	–	17 %

Saturated and Polyunsaturated Fatty Acids

The difference between saturated and mono- and polyunsaturated fatty acids has to do with the chemical structure of the fats. Depending on how many carbon and hydrogen atoms are present in the fatty acid molecule (which consists of a long chain of atoms) and in what form of bond they exist (single or double bond), a distinction is made between these three types of fatty acid. For general consumption, it is important to know that two or all three of these different forms of fatty acid are usually contained in food fats (including plant fats). Evening primrose oil, for example, contains, in addition to the polyunsaturated essential fatty acids of linoleic and gamma-linolenic acid, the monounsaturated oil acid and the saturated fatty acids of stearic and palmitic acid.

Fatty acids consist of carbon, hydrogen, and oxygen. When the binding capacity of oxygen and hydrogen atoms to carbon has not been fully exhausted, the terms "monounsaturated" and "polyunsaturated" are used to describe the fatty acids. These unsaturated fatty acids are invaluable to the functioning of the body because they are absorbed so easily.

Which Fats Are Good for Our Health and Which Are Not?

In principle, the following applies: All essential fatty acids—that is to say, all vitally important fatty acids that cannot be produced by the body—are always polyunsaturated. Yet not all polyunsaturated fatty acids are essential. The more unsaturated fatty acids are contained in a fat, the thinner it becomes. Saturated fatty acids, on the other hand, which are predominantly derived from animal fats and are considered to be unhealthy because they elevate the cholesterol level among other effects, help to solidify fats. Butter and lard as well as coconut fat are relatively hard—they contain highly saturated fatty acids.

The body burns these fats and obtains energy from them. Superfluous fat that is not burned will be deposited as stored fat, and in due time this may result in being overweight. The body doesn't care whether it uses plant or animal fats as an energy source. As a rule, however, plant fats contain a distinctly higher portion of unsaturated and essential fatty acids than animal fats, so they are more easily digested and much better for us.

Overview of Edible Fats

Edible Fat	Saturated Fatty Acids	Monounsaturated Fatty Acids	Polyunsaturated Fatty Acids
Cottonseed oil	25 %	25 %	50 %
Butter	64 %	33 %	3 %
Peanut oil	19 %	50 %	31 %
Herring oil	22 %	56 %	22 %
Coconut oil	92 %	6 %	2 %
Corn oil	17 %	32 %	51 %
Olive oil	19 %	73 %	8 %
Palm kernel oil	83 %	15 %	2 %
Palm oil	46 %	44 %	10 %
Rape seed oil	8 %	60 %	32 %
Beef suet	52 %	44 %	4 %
Safflower oil	14 %	24 %	62 %
Pork lard	41 %	49 %	10 %
Soybean oil	14 %	24 %	62 %
Sunflower oil	8 %	27 %	65 %

In the consumption of edible fats, you should always watch for a balance between saturated, monounsaturated, and polyunsaturated fatty acids. An optimally balanced diet would consist of one-third saturated and monounsaturated and of two-thirds polyunsaturated fatty acids.

Recommended Daily Dosage of Fatty Acids

❧ In order to prevent a deficiency in polyunsaturated essential fatty acids, an adult should consume approximately 10 grams of them per day.

❧ Children require even more of them during their growing phase. Their daily minimum requirement should therefore be more than 10 grams.

❧ For comparison, 3 teaspoons of safflower, soybean, or sunflower oil contain 10 grams of polyunsaturated essential fatty acids.

❧ Highly polyunsaturated fatty acids are also found in borage, hemp, black currant, black caraway, and gooseberry oil.

Absorption of Linoleic Acid

The form of linoleic acid that can be utilized by the body and is present in evening primrose oil is biologically active. In their chemical structure, biologically active fatty acids represent the natural, unchanged composition. Through the artificial processing of these fatty acids, such as in the production of many types of margarine or qualitatively low-grade food oils, the biologically active fatty acids can be converted into biologically inactive, transmissible fatty acids. Transmissible fatty acids occur in animal fats in small amounts. In the production of margarine, for example, they occur when the plant fats harden. If the biologically active linoleic acid is changed into a transmissible configuration through certain industrial processing procedures, the enzyme delta-6-desaturase can no longer convert it. As hard as the busy little enzyme might try, it wastes its energy on the transmissible configuration without being able to convert the linoleic acid into the valuable gamma-linolenic acid.

Margarine has been much maligned among experts as being one of the main suppliers of transmissible fatty acids. It must be mentioned in all fairness, though, that with the help of modern production processes the portion of transmissible fatty acids in high-grade market products has been reduced to below 10 percent.

Hidden Transmissible Fatty Acids in Food

American tests have shown that transmissible fatty acids are partially hidden in many foods—among them foremost in margarine.

Foods	Portion of Transmissible Fatty Acids
Sweets	Up to 38.6 %
Baked goods	Up to 38.5 %
French fries	Up to 37.4 %
Vegetable oils for frying	Up to 37.3 %
Hard types of margarine	Up to 36.0 %
Soft types of margarine	Up to 21.3 %
Diet margarine	Up to 17.9 %
Low-grade vegetable oils	Up to 13.7 %

Production of Gamma-Linolenic Acid

The body produces the important gamma-linolenic acid from linoleic acid, or more precisely from biologically active linoleic acid, meaning the natural form, as it is present in evening primrose oil. This in turn is the basic substance for prostaglandin, any of various unsaturated fatty acids that take part in nearly all processes and chemical reactions in the body. If there is a deficiency of gamma-linolenic acid, this can result in physical consequences ranging from a diminished feeling of well-being all the way to possibly serious illnesses. However, such consequences can be prevented by taking the oil made from the seeds of evening primrose.

Interference in the Production of Gamma-Linolenic Acid

In order to produce gamma-linolenic acid from linoleic acid, the enzyme delta-6-desaturase is required. This very active but also extremely fragile enzyme makes this metabolic process possible. There are several factors, such as diseases or other harmful influences having to do with lifestyle, that may impede or even significantly diminish this process. These are some examples:

❦ Hereditary predisposition
❦ Diabetes mellitus
❦ Viral infections
❦ Advanced age
❦ Excessive consumption of alcohol
❦ Smoking
❦ Lack of exercise
❦ Psychological pressure, due to constant stress
❦ Elevated cholesterol level, due to a high consumption of animal fats
❦ Consumption of too many saturated and hardened fats
❦ Excessive consumption of transmissible fatty acids
❦ Zinc deficiency, due to faulty or unbalanced nutrition

Linoleic acid is found in sunflower, thistle, and corn oil, for example. Linolenic acid is contained in rape seed, soybean, and linseed oil.

It is true that the oil made from borage seeds contains more gamma-linolenic acid than evening primrose oil, but its other ingredients are not without controversy.

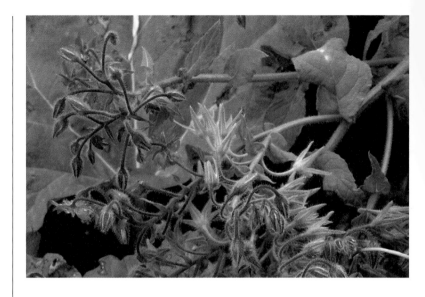

Along with relieving the itching in cases of dry skin due to eczema, the therapeutic effects of gamma-linolenic acid include longer periods of symptom-free phases and therefore possibly less of a need to take additional medication.

Why Should We Use Evening Primrose Oil?

Because gamma-linolenic acid is so important for the production of prostaglandin in the body, the following question naturally arises: Why shouldn't we use oils with a higher content of this fatty acid, such as the oil made from the seeds of currants or borage oil?

Linoleic Acid and Gamma-Linolenic Acid

The answer lies in the fact that evening primrose oil contains both fatty acids—linoleic acid and gamma-linolenic acid. Consequently, it can be said that we use a two-pronged approach:

❧ The body receives the basic agent of linoleic acid from which it can manufacture the needed gamma-linolenic acid on its own.

❧ If this step should be impaired through certain obstructing factors, the body will be able to also absorb the gamma-linolenic acid directly.

Prostaglandin

Prostaglandin (PG) perform a variety of hormonelike actions. Although true hormones are produced in various glands of the body and then moved by the bloodstream to their intended places of use, such as the digestive tract, prostaglandin are produced directly in the tissue—that is, in the location where they are needed. Also, prostaglandin are not produced and then stored. They are produced only at the time when they are needed; then, after they take effect, they are immediately expelled. They are therefore short-lived yet highly active.

More than thirty different types of prostaglandin are known today, and they are divided into the following three groups: PG1, PG2, and PG3. Gamma-linolenic acid, as it is present in evening primrose oil, is the basic substance of the prostaglandin in groups 1 and 2.

Prostaglandin, by the way, are not associated with the prostate. They were merely labeled as such back in the thirties, when Svante von Euler-Chelpin, a Swedish neurologist (1905–1983), who also received the Nobel prize in medicine, first discovered them in the seminal fluid of sheep. He assumed that prostaglandin were formed in the prostate, but this hypothesis soon proved to be in error because prostaglandin are found in nearly all the organs of both men and women. The name, however, was retained.

Cold-pressed oils made from various plants contain many vitamins and natural fatty acids, but they are less durable in comparison to oils extracted through pressings under elevated temperatures.

How the Prostaglandin in Group 1 Work

After gamma-linolenic acid has been produced in the body from linoleic acid, the next step is the production of a substance called dihomo-gamma-linolenic acid, from which the various prostaglandin in group 1, among them prostaglandin E1, are formed. Prostaglandin E1 plays an important controlling role in a number of metabolic processes in the body. If there is a deficiency in prostaglandin E1, an illness will inevitably result.

Unsaturated fatty acids feed the cell membrane, which protects the cell nucleus and the inner portion of the cell. They also insulate the nerve cells, lower the harmful LDL-cholesterol level, and guard against coronaries, strokes, and arteriosclerosis.

Functions of Prostaglandin E1

❦ Controls the routing of nerve impulses through the nerve paths and, at the nerve-path endings, the release of chemical messengers for further information relays via the bloodstream

❦ Regulates and coordinates the functioning of the brain

❦ Controls and supports the immune system

❦ Activates T-lymphocytes, which act as defense cells against pathogens that may have invaded the body

❦ Reinforces the effect of insulin in the metabolism of sugar

❦ Lowers the cholesterol level

❦ Stimulates the burning of fat in the body

❦ Helps to remove excessive weight

❦ Strengthens the effect of adenosine monophosphate, a substance that translates the messages relayed through hormones from the exterior wall of the cell to the interior of the cell and is responsible for the smooth functioning of the muscles

❦ Controls the transport of calcium through the body

❦ Stimulates the gastric mucous membrane to help protect the lining of the stomach from the aggressive gastric acid

❦ Prevents withdrawal symptoms in alcohol-dependent individuals and supports the regeneration of the liver

❦ Counteracts skin infections

❦ Prevents thromboses

❦ Helps keep coronary vessels open

❦ Stops the formation of blood clots

❦ Lowers blood pressure

❦ Lessens the release of tissue-damaging substances during infections of the body

❦ Lowers inflammation-producing substances in rheumatic diseases and arthritis, and promotes the healing of such inflammations

❦ Protects against arteriosclerosis

❦ Controls the activity of female sex hormones and regulates the menstrual cycle

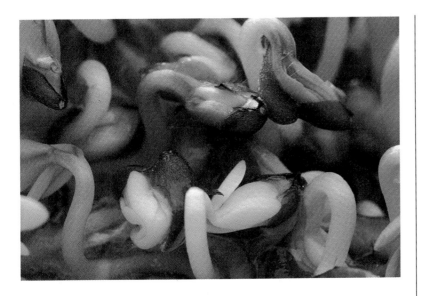

Sprouts, such as wheat, cress, and soybean, contain a great deal of vitamin B6 and are especially easy to digest.

Production of Dihomo-Gamma-Linolenic Acid

In order to form dihomo-gamma-linolenic acid from gamma-linolenic acid, the body requires water-soluble vitamin B6 (pyridoxine), which is contained in the following foods.

Foods Rich in Vitamin B6

Broccoli, cauliflower, green beans, brussels sprouts, kohlrabi, bananas, leeks, tomatoes, bell peppers, a variety of sprouts, wheat germ, yeast, soybeans, brown rice, lentils, avocados, sardines, salmon, poultry, calves' liver, beef, and pork.

Production of Prostaglandin E1

In order to then be able to produce the valuable prostaglandin E1 from dihomo-gamma-linolenic acid, the water-soluble vitamins C (ascorbic acid) and niacin (nicotine acid) as well as the trace element zinc are required. These too can be ingested through food.

Fats protect the body from mechanical effects and cold. They are the suppliers of energy, a component of the cell membrane, the primary component of biological substances, and carriers of aromatic substances, as well as a transport medium for fat-soluble vitamins.

Foods Rich in Vitamin C

Citrus fruit, black currants, rose hips, red berries, strawberries, kiwi fruit, papayas, nectarines, broccoli, kohlrabi, cauliflower, brussels sprouts, cabbage, potatoes, spinach, and bell peppers.

Foods Rich in Niacin

Niacin is contained in certain foods but can also be formed in the body from tryptophan, an amino acid. The following foods contain either niacin or tryptophan: lean beef and pork, organ meats (such as kidneys, heart, and liver), sardines, shrimp, roast chicken, peas, apricots, wheat germ, mushrooms, peanuts, and coffee.

Foods Rich in Zinc

Oysters, lamb, beef, veal, chicken, turkey, tuna, shrimp, mussels, wheat and rye germ, barley, oat flakes, cheese, pumpkin seeds, sunflower seeds, sesame seeds, lentils, peas, and onions.

Medications that contain acetyl-salicylic acid (ASA) prevent the conversion of arachidonic acid into the prostaglandin of group 2. In this way, they contribute to lowering fever and decreasing pain.

Prostaglandin in Group 2

The prostaglandin in group 2 are also formed from dihomo-gamma-linolenic acid. However, this takes place with the help of arachidonic acid, which enables the cells of the body to remain elastic. Arachidonic acid is produced in all living beings and then stored in cells. When the cell walls threaten to become too rigid, the acid is released in order to make them elastic again. When there is a source of inflammation in the body, the prostaglandin from group 2 are produced from the arachidonic acid. Pain and fever often accompany inflammations. The prostaglandin of group 2 are also capable of lowering blood pressure and supporting the muscular activity of the uterus during childbirth.

Inflammations Resulting from Improper Diet

Arachidonic acid, from which the prostaglandin in group 2 are formed, is contained in all foods derived from animals. If it is ingested in amounts beyond normal food intake, the prostaglandin from group 2 will increasingly be produced. The human metabolism develops a substance besides arachidonic acid that promotes a progression of the inflammation: the eucosanoids.

Stopping Inflammations with Correct Diet

If there are any sources of inflammation in the body, the unpleasant symptoms can be influenced positively through a special diet. The amount of prostaglandin from groups 1 and 2 will shift as a result of a change in diet in favor of the prostaglandin from group 1, which counteract the inflammation processes. With the help of this diet, even inflammations in the joints occurring with the presence of rheumatoid illnesses, and therefore also the accompanying pain, can be lessened considerably and will sometimes even disappear altogether. Professor Olaf Adam of the Orthopedic Hospital in München-Harlaching, Germany, says, "Many patients who otherwise would have to take medications for the rest of their lives can dramatically reduce their intake of medications or even do without them completely if they follow a diet designed for rheumatism."

An effective diet for rheumatism requires patience and perseverance. According to Professor Olaf Adam, "It will take a minimum of six weeks of consistently watching one's food intake before an improvement will be noticed."

Anti-inflammation Diet Guidelines

❦ Eat no more than two small meat servings per week.

❦ Use high-grade plant fats in food preparation, such as walnut, flax, hemp seed, soybean, or rape seed oil.

❦ Include in your daily diet plenty of fruit and vegetables that have been carefully prepared in order to preserve the maximum amount of vitamins and trace elements.

❦ Eat meals prepared from soybeans or fish (preferably mackerel, herring, or ocean salmon) at least twice a week.

❦ Reduce your alcohol consumption to a minimum.

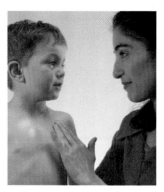

Evening primrose oil: a good means of prevention and healing even for children

Prevention and Healing with Evening Primrose Oil

Evening primrose oil can be a gentle aid in the presence of many health problems, and it can even prevent some. It also promotes a sense of well-being, alleviating the harmful effects of stress or removing them altogether. When taken during pregnancy, evening primrose oil can help significantly in the prevention of later allergies in children.

Alcohol Dependency

Alcoholism, now regarded as a disease, can be defined as an overwhelming desire to drink alcohol, even though it causes harm. Alcohol is a drug, and, in the United States, alcoholism is the most widespread form of drug abuse, affecting nearly five million people. Half of all fatal car accidents each year in the United States are due to drunk drivers, and drinking is a major cause of financial, social, and personal problems—to say nothing of severe health problems. In fact, roughly 15 percent of heavy drinkers in the United States develop cirrhosis, a disease of the liver that can be fatal.

Alcohol and Evening Primrose Oil

Moderate alcohol consumption reinforces the positive effect of prostaglandin E1, which is derived from evening primrose oil. However, excessive alcohol consumption blocks its effect. An excess of alcohol also blocks the production of gamma-linolenic acid from biologically active linoleic acid. Tests on alcoholics have further shown that their prostaglandin E1 level was very low. This represents a considerable risk factor in the incidence of heart diseases, liver ailments, high blood pressure, general immune deficiency, and functional impairments of the brain and nerve cells.

Evening Primrose Oil Supports Withdrawal

Once alcoholics have decided to stop drinking, evening primrose oil can help them remain sober because it reduces the craving for alcohol. It also lessens the dreaded withdrawal symptoms, such as trembling and depressions, while supporting the regeneration of the functions of the brain and liver cells.

Evening Primrose Oil Prevents Hangovers

Salads or cold snacks prepared with 1 or 2 teaspoons of evening primrose oil (per person) can prevent headaches and other hangover symptoms from occurring the following day. Four to six 500 mg capsules of evening primrose oil taken at bedtime after an evening of drinking will have the same effect.

Allergies in Children

Allergic dermatitis is the most common skin condition in American children younger than ten years old. Ten percent of American children are diagnosed with it now, as opposed to 3 percent during the sixties. Eight percent of American children younger than six years old have some form of food intolerance, and of this group 2 to 4 percent have food allergies. Doctors are afraid that these figures will not come down in the future, but that the incidence of allergies will continue to increase among young children.

"Asthma, hay fever, and neurodermatitis will be the epidemics of the twenty-first century. The peak of these illnesses has not been reached by far," says Professor Ulrich Wahn, an allergy specialist at Virchow Hospital in Berlin. In cases of asthma and neuro-dermatitis, both of which are types of allergic reaction, evening primrose oil can help significantly in alleviating discomfort.

Are Allergies Hereditary?

According to studies, children suffer from allergies more frequently when their parents are also allergic. If one parent is allergic, the probability of his or her offspring also suffering from allergies is 40 percent. When both parents have a history of allergies, that risk climbs to 60 percent.

How an Allergy Starts

The catalysts for an allergy include pollen, house dust, animal hair, mold spores, ingredients in food, and insecticides, as well as chemicals in the air, in cleaning agents, in cosmetics, in furniture, and in other materials. In each of these instances, an immune system that has gone awry reassesses basically harmless substances as dangerous. An overcompensating immune reaction follows, during which inflammation-promoting substances are produced. The symptoms range from hay fever, which in every third case will develop into asthma within ten years, to skin eczema (neurodermatitis, also referred to as atopic eczema), all the way to nausea, vomiting, stomach and intestinal cramps, and diarrhea.

Causes of Allergies in Toddlers

Excessive cleanliness during the first years of life may increase the risk of children becoming allergic. This is how German scientists at the Clinic for Childhood and Youth Medicine at the University of Bochum explain it: A child's early contact with pathogens, such as bacteria and viruses, may actually stabilize the immune system so that later allergies don't develop. Therefore, parents need to be mindful that their children are not growing up in an overly hygienic and too clean environment.

Normal provisions of cleanliness in the care of infants and toddlers may prevent later problems from arising from allergies.

Causes of Allergies in Infants

In addition to a number of other influences—such as environmental pollution, for example—there are two important factors that contribute to the incidence of allergies in infants:

❧ When the functioning of the enzyme delta-6-desaturase, which is required for the conversion of linoleic acid into gamma-linolenic acid, is partially impaired, this leads to a deficiency of gamma-linolenic acid. This in turn leads to an insufficient production of prostaglandin E1, the protection factor in allergies.

❧ Breast milk also contains gamma-linolenic acid. It constitutes about 1 percent of the fat content in breast milk. When babies cannot be nursed, this can result in a deficiency of gamma-linolenic acid and therefore also a deficiency of the allergy-preventing prostaglandin E1.

How Mothers Can Prevent Allergies

Mothers Who Nurse

Studies have shown that mothers who took evening primrose oil during the second and sixth months of nursing increased the content of gamma-linolenic acid in their breast milk. Mothers can therefore contribute toward making sure that their babies will receive a sufficient supply of gamma-linolenic acid for the production of the allergy-protection factor contained in prostaglandin E1. This is especially important for mothers who themselves suffer from allergies. They most likely have a lack of gamma-linolenic acid in their bodies, which also affects the content of gamma-linolenic acid in their breast milk.

Mothers Who Don't Nurse

It is important to directly administer the valuable gamma-linolenic acid to babies who are not nursing as well as to toddlers. A baby's digestive system is not yet fully developed during its first five months of life, so the gamma-linolenic acid can be absorbed only partially through the intestinal tract. Even toddlers, whose digestive systems are fully developed, were observed to have difficulties absorbing gamma-linolenic acid. It is therefore recommended to massage evening primrose oil directly into the skin of infants and toddlers. The oil is then quickly absorbed into the body. In establishing a dosage, it's best to go by the amount of gamma-linolenic acid that is normally contained in the breast milk of healthy mothers. This amount corresponds to approximately 1,500 milligrams of evening primrose oil.

In contrast to the milk produced by most other mammals, human breast milk contains gamma-linolenic acid. Even cow's milk contains only linoleic acid, and not gamma-linolenic acid.

Asthma

Nearly fifteen million people in the United States suffer from self-reported asthma with agonizing coughing spells and difficulty breathing. This is an increase of approximately five million people since 1990. The illness is generally underestimated—in fact, in the United States among asthmatics five to twenty-four years of age, the asthma death rate almost doubled from 1980 to 1993.

Organic Causes of Asthma

Asthma is caused by a spasm of the bronchial musculature together with an inflammation of the bronchial tubes, a swelling of the mucous membranes, and an excessive output of mucus. Due to the spasms, the used air cannot be exhaled completely, so there is insufficient space in the lungs when fresh air is inhaled again. What follow are the feeling of not getting enough air and a difficulty in breathing, even though the inhaling is actually less impaired than the exhaling.

In their examinations of asthma patients, doctors in England discovered that the fatty acid profile, or the presence of various fatty acids in their patients, deviated from the norm. They suspect a connection between these fatty acid abnormalities and the onset of asthma.

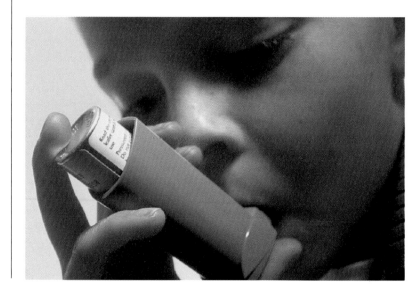

A controversial, instant aid for acute asthma attacks: an inhaler with a spray that dilates the bronchial passages

What Makes Evening Primrose Oil Effective against Asthma?

In the event of an asthma attack, leukotriene are also involved. These substances are formed from arachidonic acid, and the enzyme 5-lipoxygenase plays a part as well. Gamma-linolenic acid, as it is contained in evening primrose oil, is capable of curbing the production of leukotriene and thereby contributes to the successful prevention of asthma attacks. In addition, prostaglandin E1, which is formed in the body from gamma-linolenic acid, also assists in preventing the release of arachidonic acid, which is stored in the cells of the body. Gamma-linolenic acid thus reduces the amount of the original component from which leukotriene are produced. At the same time, prostaglandin E1, the tissue hormone, has an anti-inflammatory effect.

In cases of allergic asthma, the allergens should be avoided as much as possible insofar as they are known.

A Tea with Evening Primrose Oil for Treating Asthma

A tea made from ibis roots with the addition of evening primrose oil has a calming, anticonvulsive effect on asthma attacks. Mix 1 tablespoon of ibis root in 1 cup of cold water, and allow to sit for half an hour. Drain and stir. Heat to about 95 to 104°F (35 to 40°C). Mix 15 drops of evening primrose oil with 1 tablespoon of tea, and add to the tea. Drink 1 cup of this in small sips at night.

Ibis roots, which are used in the preparation of teas, are available at special herb stores, natural food stores, and certain drugstores.

What Else You Can Do

❦ See to it that you get sufficient physical exercise. Try to pursue endurance sports, such as hiking, bicycling, swimming, or cross-country skiing.

❦ It would be best to forego nicotine altogether.

❦ Keep your weight under control.

❦ Try to learn relaxation techniques, such as visualizations or specific breathing exercises.

❦ Help prevent infections with sauna treatments or alternating hot-and-cold showers.

Breast Disorders (Mastopathies)

Every second woman on an average goes through phases during which she suffers from a generally painful but benign disorder of the breast (mastopathy). Some women even suffer all the time from this condition. Hormonal changes during the menstrual cycle are responsible for these benign changes in the breast tissue. The problems usually show up during the week prior to the menstrual period, when small nodules in the breasts can be felt and the breasts swell up and are painful and extremely sensitive. Once the period begins, the symptoms lessen. The symptoms increase with age, reaching their climax when women are in their forties; then they gradually decrease after the onset of menopause until they disappear altogether. There are essentially two forms of this benign breast condition:

❦ A cystic mastopathy is present in about 75 percent of all cases. Cysts form in the glandular tissue (small cavities) and fill with liquid.

❦ In rarer cases, there is no presence of cysts filled with liquid but rather a hardening of the connective tissue. This condition is called fibroadenoma.

Results of Studies

Several studies have shown that benign breast diseases can be treated very successfully with evening primrose oil:

❦ At Western General Hospital in Edinburgh, Scotland, 566 women with benign breast diseases were observed over a period of seven years. Those patients who were treated with evening primrose oil in combination with vitamin B6 showed a significant improvement in their symptoms.

❦ At the University Clinic in Manchester, Great Britain, 75 percent of all women with pain in their breasts were treated successfully with evening primrose oil.

❦ Doctors at the University of Wales in Cardiff discovered in blood tests of women suffering from mastopathy that they showed an

A study that originated at King's College Hospital in London and was conducted all over Great Britain with 276 physicians participating investigated the treatment methods of patients diagnosed with mastopathies. The study revealed that 30 percent of the physicians obtained good results with a treatment of evening primrose oil.

Never Neglect Cancer Prevention!

Before you decide to take evening primrose oil, your gynecologist should absolutely rule out any possibility of changes in the breast tissue being due to malignant cell growth. Because there is also a slightly increased risk of breast cancer in patients suffering from mastopathy, all nodules should be monitored carefully over the course of regular examinations for cancer prevention.

excess in saturated fatty acids and a deficiency in essential fatty acids. When evening primrose oil was prescribed to these women, the relationship of the fatty acids was normalized. A further study indicated that in cases of mastopathy a treatment with evening primrose oil was equal to treatments with chemical substances that affect the hormonal output—but without the side effects occasionally caused by such medications, such as nausea, backache, weight gain, dizziness, skin eczema, and reddening of the skin.

Evening Primrose Oil in the Treatment of Breast Disorders

Various studies have concluded that an excess of the hormone prolactin and a lack of prostaglandin E1 are responsible for the formation of cysts in the breast tissue. Both conditions can be influenced successfully through the ingestion of evening primrose oil.

The best results in the treatment of mastopathy have been obtained when two 500 mg capsules of evening primrose oil are taken three times daily. However, this treatment does require some patience. The problems do not disappear immediately, but only diminish gradually. The full success of the treatment can only be seen after three months of therapy.

If you suffer from mastopathy, you should avoid all beverages containing caffeine, such as coffee, tea, and soft drinks, because they lead to an increased concentration of prolactin in the breast tissue.

Cancer

Laboratory tests indicate that the gamma-linolenic acid produced in the body from evening primrose oil and the metabolically derived prostaglandin E1 have an extremely positive effect in the battle against cancer.

Evening Primrose Oil: The New Anti-cancer Drug?

It is still not entirely clear through what mechanism the prostaglandin E1 formed from evening primrose oil succeeds in reducing cancer cells. But it has been possible to determine that cancer cells—contrary to healthy cells—have lost the ability to convert linoleic acid into gamma-linolenic acid. Although they produce large quantities of prostaglandin E2, they no longer produce any prostaglandin E1. One hypothesis holds that the degeneration of benign cells into cancerous cells runs parallel to the loss in the capacity to produce prostaglandin E1. Therefore, it is believed that this development could be reversed if the cancer cells received prostaglandin E1 from an exterior source.

Men who consume mostly unsaturated fats, such as those found in evening primrose oil, have been seen to contract prostate cancer at a below-average rate. When evening primrose oil is used in the prepa-

The effectiveness of evening primrose oil with regard to cancer is still much disputed among scientists. It is certainly not a miracle drug. However, numerous tests give rise to the hope that this natural substance may be quite beneficial in conjunction with other means of cancer treatment.

Evening Primrose Oil Put to the Test

❦ Researchers at the Medical University of South Africa treated animal and human cancer cells with gamma-linolenic acid in the laboratory and discovered that the cancer growth receded by 70 percent.

❦ Scientists at Nizam's Institute in Hyderabad, India, obtained similar results. They discovered that the linoleic and gamma-linolenic acid in evening primrose oil can bind certain proteins that otherwise stimulate the formation and growth of cancerous cells.

Animal Fats and Prostate Cancer

In an ongoing study conducted with 51,000 men participating since 1986, scientists at Harvard Medical School have discovered that men who eat a diet rich in animal fats run an 80 percent increased risk of contracting prostate cancer. Although the animal fats do not directly trigger the cancer, they speed up its development and promote the conversion of harmless growths into malignant tumors.

ration of cold foods, the body ingests gamma-linolenic acid, which protects against cancer. It is therefore conceivable that a diet that includes evening primrose oil may drastically reduce the risk of contracting prostate cancer.

The Application of Evening Primrose Oil as a Preventive against Cancer

Green tea lowers the risk of contracting stomach, lung, or liver cancer. This was discovered by scientists at the University of California at Berkeley. Therefore, it is believed that the effect of green tea could be combined with the general potential of evening primrose oil as a preventive treatment against cancer.

Pour 1 cup of hot water over 1 teaspoon of green tea. Let the tea steep for 10 minutes, and strain. Allow the tea to cool down to 95°F (35°C). Put 20 drops of evening primrose oil into a shot glass, and mix with 1 tablespoon of milk. Add this mixture to the green tea. You will obtain an optimal effect in the prevention of cancer if you drink one cup of this tea per day.

Recipes for dishes with evening primrose oil are found in the recipe section, starting on page 82.

Many scientists see a connection between diets containing excessive amounts of saturated fatty acids derived from animal fats and denatured vegetable oils, and the huge increase in heart and circulatory diseases and certain forms of cancer.

Chronic Fatigue Syndrome (CFS)

Constant states of fatigue are often disregarded. But, in connection with allergies, fungal infections, headaches, and pains in the joints and the extremities, they can actually be a symptom of chronic fatigue syndrome (CFS). In the United States, it is estimated that half a million people suffer from a CFS-like condition. In individual cases, an improvement of CFS has been seen after treatment with evening primrose oil, although no scientific proof exists at this time. At the University of Miami, one patient was treated successfully with evening primrose oil and vitamin B12. A similar result following treatment with evening primrose oil and vitamin B12 was reported by a patient group diagnosed with CFS in New Zealand.

Diabetes Mellitus

Type I diabetes (also known as juvenile diabetes or insulin-dependent diabetes mellitus) may already occur in newborns; their bodies produce too little insulin or none at all. Type II diabetes (often called adult-onset diabetes or non-insulin-dependent diabetes mellitus) is usually due not only to a lack of insulin but also to a reduced reaction of the cells to this hormone.

About 5 percent of the American population either have or will have diabetes mellitus, a chronic disorder of the sugar metabolism. Along with the already unpleasant enough symptoms of diabetes, there is the added danger of serious secondary effects due to the long-term increase in the level of blood sugar.

Sugar is absorbed in the form of carbohydrates through food, such as fruit, pasta, bread, and potatoes. The carbohydrates are turned into glucose in the intestinal tract. The glucose is then temporarily stored in the liver, which regularly delivers it into the bloodstream. The bloodstream in turn transports the glucose to each cell of the body, where it is burned. Because the cells cannot open up by themselves in order to absorb the glucose, insulin, the pancreatic hormone, intervenes by guiding the glucose into the nuclei of the cells.

Organic Causes of Diabetes Mellitus

If the body produces too little insulin or if it is limited in its effectiveness, glucose cannot be transported to the cells of the body in order

Symptoms of Diabetes Mellitus

❧ Excessive thirst, even without physical exertion, and frequent urination

❧ Constant fatigue, weariness, inability to concentrate

❧ Unpleasant itching extending over the whole body, but especially in the genital area

❧ Poor and prolonged healing of wounds, infection of even small and superficial skin injuries

❧ Tendency to form furuncles, small knots at the hair roots that then become infected and erupt in pustules

❧ Frequent episodes of neuritis

❧ Increasingly lowered sex drive

❧ Excessive perspiration, even at rest

❧ Feelings of ravenous hunger, nausea after eating

❧ Muscle spasms, pronounced trembling of the fingers

Doctors at Children's Hospital of Juntendo University in Tokyo administered gamma-linolenic acid in the form of evening primrose oil to eleven diabetic children (Type I diabetes) over a duration of four months. At the end of this period, they found that the metabolism of the prostaglandin and the lipometabolism had improved and stabilized through the direct administration of gamma-linolenic acid.

to be burned. This leads to an increase in the blood-sugar level—in other words, the patient suffers from diabetes mellitus.

The Two Forms of Diabetes Mellitus

Juvenile, or Type I, Diabetes

It is possible that the pancreas already during youth will produce less and less insulin and, in some cases, even cease to produce any at all. Roughly 10 percent of all diabetics fall into the category of Type I diabetes. They must add the insulin hormone for the rest of their lives by means of injections.

Adult-Onset, or Type II, Diabetes

This form usually occurs after age forty. Eating too many foods rich in fats together with a lack of exercise have damaged the body over

Colorful seducers: Candy is pure poison for diabetics.

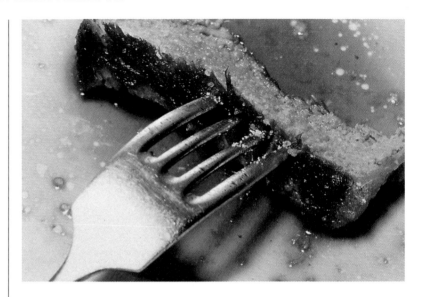

the years to such an extent that it no longer responds sufficiently to insulin. If there is a predisposition, the risk increases. It lies at roughly 40 percent if there is a family history of diabetes mellitus. Because the production of insulin in Type II diabetics is reduced gradually over a longer period of time, they rarely require insulin injections and when they do, this is usually only necessary in advanced age. Normally, a restricted diet will be sufficient to prevent a worsening of the condition and the outbreak of secondary symptoms.

Secondary Illnesses Related to Diabetes Mellitus

Neuropathy

Diabetes mellitus damages the nerves so that the speed with which nerve impulses are conducted is decreased, which then leads to a gradually increasing loss of feeling. First indications for this are a tingling sensation, like a feeling of ants crawling along the extremities. Later on, this may lead to complete numbness. Neuropathy is also the reason why injuries to the toes are not noticed, even when the injuries have progressed to the point where tissue dies. Diabetics cannot feel a warning pain in these instances.

Micro-angiopathy

Due to an impaired sugar metabolism, protein deposits will tend to form on the interior walls of small vessels. The already small diameters of the vessels will be restricted even further, with circulatory problems as a result. A symptom of this may be the impaired healing of wounds.

Macro-angiopathy

Fat deposits will form even on the inner walls of larger vessels, which will gradually become more and more restricted. This may manifest itself in serious circulatory problems—for example, in the legs—but may also lead to a heart attack or a stroke.

Retinopathy

The dangerous consequences of diabetes on the blood vessels also affect the blood vessels in the eyes, which become fragile and brittle. Small dilations form, and they will erupt and lead to a bleeding into the retina or the lens. The body tries to repair such damages and to close the injury with connective tissue. In order to secure the circulation in the eye, new blood vessels are formed at the same time. The result is an increasing dimness of vision, gradually limiting the ability to see, until total blindness sets in.

Nephropathy

Damage to the vessels in the kidneys gradually leads to a decreased functioning of them all the way to total kidney failure. At the point when the kidneys can no longer fulfill their detoxifying function, the patient will have to undergo dialysis treatments.

Scientific Studies

Two English studies on more than 400 patients suffering from diabetes who had been treated with gamma-linolenic acid showed that the symptoms of nerve damage associated with diabetes mellitus were significantly reduced. Observations by Andrew J. M. Boulton at

Type II diabetics, in particular, who usually are overweight, do not get enough exercise, and have high levels of blood fat due to their rich diets, are frequently affected by macro-angiopathy.

Doctors at Metropolitan Geriatric Hospital in Tokyo found that a daily dosage of 4 grams of evening primrose oil, combined with 2.4 grams of sardine oil and 200 milligrams of vitamin E, successfully lowered the elevated blood-fat levels in diabetics and helped in the prevention of vascular occlusions. A noticeable improvement was seen after only four weeks. This was accompanied by a slight weight loss, which is extremely important for most diabetics.

Royal Hospital in Manchester, Great Britain, noted similar results. Dr. Boulton had prescribed a daily dosage of 480 mg of gamma-linolenic acid to 146 diabetics over the course of one year. Measurements of nerve conductivity showed an improvement over values that had been obtained prior to the ingestion of gamma-linolenic acid.

How Evening Primrose Oil Prevents Serious Effects of Diabetes

Due to the blocking of the enzyme delta-6-desaturase, the conversion of linoleic acid into gamma-linolenic acid is disrupted. Yet gamma-linolenic acid is the basic substance for the production of prostaglandin E1, which protects the vessels and prevents fat deposits from forming on their interior walls. Prostaglandin E1 keeps the blood thin at the same time and thereby counteracts the circulatory problems characteristic of diabetes mellitus. Additionally, prostaglandin E1 can stimulate the activity of the insulin still present in the body. This makes it possible to balance the pancreatic hormone deficiency.

When evening primrose oil is ingested, the conversion step from linoleic to gamma-linolenic acid becomes unnecessary because the latter is present in evening primrose oil. Diabetics can therefore ingest this basic substance in order to promote the production of prostaglandin E1.

Dryness in the Mouth and the Eyes

Dryness in the mouth and the eyes is a rare syndrome that frequently coincides with arthritis. In this disorder, the production of fluid by the saliva glands of the mouth and the tear glands of the eyes is reduced. The patients will suffer from an excessively dry mouth as well as a burning, scratchy sensation in the eyes. Various clinical studies have demonstrated that these symptoms may be alleviated significantly when evening primrose oil is taken.

Elevated Cholesterol Level

Cholesterol is a fat substance that is formed in the body in part by the liver, the intestinal system, and the skin. But it is also ingested with food derived from animal fats. In normal concentrations, cholesterol is vital to our well-being.

The Functions of Cholesterol in the Body

🐚 Cholesterol protects the liver from illnesses, such as infections.
🐚 It is the basic substance in the production of sex and adrenocortical hormones.
🐚 Cholesterol plays a decisive part in the immune system by activating the body's power of resistance.
🐚 It promotes the absorption of vitamins A, E, and D, as well as potassium from the foods we ingest.
🐚 Cholesterol is the building substance in our red blood cells.
It provides elasticity for our muscles and makes them strong.

When Is Cholesterol Harmful?

Whether cholesterol leads to arteriosclerosis or not doesn't depend solely on its concentration in the blood. What is important is the relationship between two different cholesterol-protein combinations (lipoproteins). Cholesterol doesn't move through the body on its own but requires a transport medium, which is protein. A distinction is made between "good" and "bad" cholesterol–fat combinations.

"Bad" Lipoproteins

The LDL (low-density lipoprotein) combinations transport the cholesterol with the help of the bloodstream into the cells of the body for further processing. If there is an oversupply in the body, which results, above all, from too high an intake of animal fats in food, there will be a buildup in the vessels. This leads to the cholesterol being deposited layer by layer on the inside of the arterial walls. The result

Cholesterol is an important substance. If the body receives too little of it, this results in muscle weakness, which also affects the heart muscle and can lead to the heart stopping entirely. However, this danger is extremely low, as we ordinarily ingest more cholesterol with our food than is actually needed by the body.

An improper diet of too much meat with a high fat content can lead to the formation of arteriosclerosis.

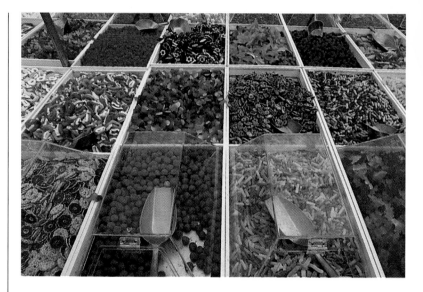

Animal fats ingested from meat, dairy products, and eggs contain mostly saturated fatty acids, which promote the harmful LDL combination. You should therefore review your consumption of such foods.

will be a progressive hardening of the arteries, which can lead to a total occlusion of the vessels.

"Good" Lipoproteins

HDL (high-density lipoprotein) combinations counteract the LDL combinations. These proteins course through the circulatory system and collect cholesterol deposits from the walls of the arteries, in order to transport them to the liver, where they will be broken down. They will be used there as the basic substance for the production of bile acid, which is necessary for digestion. If the share of the good HDL cholesterol amounts to at least a quarter of the entire cholesterol value, your health will not be endangered. Because the relationship of LDL cholesterol to HDL cholesterol also plays a part, you will have no need for concern if the total value is 300 mg per deciliter of blood, as long as the share of the good HDL cholesterol amounts to 75 mg and above per deciliter of blood. If it is below that, the risk of arteriosclerosis goes up.

How Evening Primrose Oil Lowers Cholesterol

Prostaglandin E1, which is formed in the body from the gamma-linolenic acid contained in evening primrose oil, lowers the cholesterol level. Studies have confirmed that a daily intake of eight 500 mg evening primrose oil capsules over a period of twelve weeks will lower the cholesterol level—especially the dangerous LDL-cholesterol level—by an average of 18 percent.

Recipe to Prevent High Cholesterol Levels

The substance cynarin contained in artichokes is highly effective in lowering the cholesterol level and preventing arteriosclerosis. Why not combine the healing powers of artichoke with those of evening primrose? Artichoke juice can be purchased in health food stores as a freshly pressed plant juice.

Add 1 tablespoon of artichoke juice to a glass of water, and then add 5 to 10 drops of evening primrose oil. It is even more effective if you mix the artichoke juice and the evening primrose oil with a glass of tomato juice. Tomato juice contains a great deal of vitamin B6, which the body needs in order to convert gamma-linolenic acid

Physicians at Aoto Hospital of Jikei Medical University in Tokyo administered evening primrose oil to nineteen patients with highly elevated cholesterol levels for a period of sixteen weeks and discovered that the share of the harmful LDL cholesterol decreased significantly.

Normal Cholesterol Levels

According to numerous studies conducted in the United States, the following limit levels, according to age groups, of total cholesterol in the blood—measured in mg per deciliter (mg/dl)—are recommended:

❦ To twenty-nine years of age: up to 200 mg per deciliter

❦ Thirty to thirty-nine years of age: up to 225 mg per deciliter

❦ Forty to forty-nine years of age: up to 245 mg per deciliter

❦ From fifty years of age: up to 265 mg per deciliter

into dihomo-gamma-linolenic acid, from which prostaglandin E1 is produced. It is recommended to drink one glass of this mixture twice a day.

High Cholesterol Values in Infants

Physicians at the Institute for Preventive Cardiology at the University Clinic of Hamburg, Germany, undertook an extensive study of cholesterol values in the blood of newborn infants. They found that 452 infants out of 10,000 showed significantly elevated levels of blood fat, and that these levels still had not normalized after follow-up examinations at the age of four. This was a dangerous time bomb, for high concentrations of cholesterol in the blood are the cause of coronary heart disease, which could lead to angina pectoris and even provoke a heart attack later on.

Prevention with Evening Primrose Oil

Because an analysis of the cholesterol content in the blood may not be part of the standard tests conducted for babies and children where you live, the use of evening primrose oil could be an effective preventive measure in lowering a possibly elevated cholesterol content. However, be sure to consult your physician regarding the correct dosage.

Heart Attack

Heart disease is the leading killer of Americans, claiming even more lives than cancer. It is also a leading cause of long-term disabilities. Among coronary and circulatory diseases, heart attacks rank first. In the United States, one and a half million people experience a heart attack each year. A heart attack takes place when the blood flow to the heart muscle is interrupted and the muscle begins to die.

Caution: Children who suffer from temporal lobe epilepsy should not ingest any evening primrose oil, as this could lead to a worsening of their condition. Studies have shown that this risk occurs only when a relatively high dosage of evening primrose oil is consumed, but it should still never be taken without consulting a doctor. The same applies to adults who suffer from this illness.

Watch for Early Warning Signals

A heart attack is frequently thought to come as a complete surprise. However, research at the University of Heidelberg has shown that in about 30 percent of all cases there were clear warning signals during the four weeks prior to the heart attack. They were just misinterpreted or carelessly ignored. Such signals include feelings of pressure and tightness in the chest, sometimes associated with a burning pain in back of the sternum and in the pit of the stomach. These symptoms often occur during or following physical exertion, such as sports activities, climbing stairs, or strenuous labor. Sometimes the pain will run from the stomach via the sternum into the upper arm (this occurs with the right arm more frequently than with the left) and then into the teeth of the lower jaw. Such symptoms usually disappear as soon as the physical activity ceases.

Angina Pectoris as Pre-infarct Syndrome

There is also an increased risk of a heart attack when a person suffers from unstable angina pectoris, the gradually progressive tightening of the coronary vessels. Its onset is predominantly sudden and without any warning. The attacks last longer each time and occur even during periods of minimal physical exertion or rest. Because the risk of a heart attack is highly increased during these episodes, this condi-

The cause of the early warning signals of a heart attack: At least one of the three large coronary vessels supplying the heart with blood is restricted. When physical demands are made on the body, the heart has to increase its pumping capacity, so the heart muscle must receive an increased supply of oxygen. Because this cannot be assured due to the narrowed passage, the typical symptoms will develop.

Risk Factors for a Heart Attack

- ❦ Smoking
- ❦ High blood pressure
- ❦ Stress
- ❦ Sleep apnea (breathing stops briefly during sleep at night)
- ❦ Increased cholesterol level
- ❦ Overweight
- ❦ Lack of exercise
- ❦ Genetic predisposition
- ❦ Impaired fat metabolism
- ❦ Diabetes mellitus

When a heart attack occurs, the blood circulation through at least one heart vessel is completely interrupted. Calcareous deposits, which may have been caused by a diet rich in fats, have occluded the vessel, or a blood clot has floated in from another region of the body and settled like a lid over the openings of the arteries. In both cases, the blood circulation will be interrupted. That part of the heart muscle that is supplied by this particular vessel will die from a lack of oxygen.

tion is also called pre-infarct syndrome. The highest alarm level is reached when the attacks occur after getting out of bed in the morning and last longer than 15 minutes. They are then most likely the precursors of a heart attack.

Symptoms of a Heart Attack

Sudden, very severe, and long-lasting pains in the chest in back of the sternum. The pain is often reported as a feeling of burning fire, which spreads from the chest to below the shoulder blades and sometimes also to the left arm. Pains in the right arm are rare during an acute heart attack.

❦ At the beginning of a heart attack, there is sometimes an uneasy feeling in the stomach area or upper abdomen, which over the course of one or several hours accelerates to the burning sensation described above.

❦ A pronounced feeling of pressure and tightness in the chest, together with difficulty in breathing. This feeling is often described as comparable to an iron clamp that surrounds the chest and gets tighter and tighter.

❦ Ashen, gray facial coloring, and cold perspiration on the forehead and upper lip, which is recognizable as tiny beads of perspiration.

❦ Gradually increasing feelings of restlessness and fear, which turn into panic, with mounting discomfort all the way to an overwhelming fear of dying.

❦ Nausea and sometimes vomiting.

❦ Rapid and irregular pulse, circulatory collapse, and sometimes unconsciousness.

Evening Primrose Oil as a Preventive

Hawthorn tea mixed with evening primrose oil is very suitable in the prevention of coronary diseases and deposits in the circulatory system. Prostaglandin E1, which is formed in the body from the gamma-linolenic acid contained in evening primrose oil, normalizes the cholesterol level and lowers blood pressure. The healing substances in hawthorn dilate the blood vessels and also help to stabilize blood pressure.

Pour 1 cup of hot water over 1 tablespoon of hawthorn tea (available at herbal stores and health food stores). Let stand for approximately 20 minutes, and strain. After the tea has cooled to body temperature, mix 5 to 10 drops of evening primrose oil with 1 tablespoon of cold milk and add this mixture to the tea. Drink one cup daily at bedtime.

The hawthorn tea can be sweetened with honey, according to taste. This actually enhances the heart-strengthening properties of the tea, because honey tends to lower blood pressure and also has a dilating effect on the blood vessels. In addition, honey contains the minerals potassium and magnesium, which help with circulatory problems of the heart muscle. An effective means of protection consists of 1 tablespoon of a good brand of honey per day.

You can also use fresh hawthorn juice in place of the tea. It's recommended to take 1 tablespoon of the juice mixed with 5 to 10 drops of evening primrose oil every day.

Hawthorn is a proven preventive against heart diseases stemming from arteriosclerotic changes in the coronary vessels and symptoms of wear that have to do with old age. Hawthorn is being used more and more in the follow-up treatment of heart attacks, although its importance still lies mainly in the area of prevention.

Immediate Measures in Case of a Heart Attack

When you suspect a heart attack, notify emergency immediately. It is best to let them know that this is probably a heart attack, because then the emergency crew will come equipped with specific diagnostic and emergency equipment.

❧ Allow the patient to get into a comfortable position. Loosen all restrictive clothing.

❧ Do not leave the patient alone. Try to converse quietly with the patient and to alleviate his or her fear. Do your best not to panic, yourself.

High Blood Pressure

High blood pressure is one of the leading causes of disability or death due to stroke, heart attack, heart failure, or kidney failure.

The numbers are frightening: Approximately fifty million people in the United States have high blood pressure (hypertension), which is one out of every four people. And each year, two million new cases of it are diagnosed. But most of the afflicted do not even suspect that their blood pressure has reached dangerously high levels. Consequently, they are not under a doctor's care and are in jeopardy of suffering a stroke or a heart attack as a result of their condition.

How Blood Circulation Functions

The heart pumps blood constantly through the circulatory system. In healthy people, this amounts to 5 to 6 quarts, or liters, per minute in a resting state. Under high pressure, the blood shoots from the left heart ventricle into the connecting main artery at a speed of about 27.5 inches (70 centimeters) per second. On its continuing path through the body, it will be distributed to several collateral arteries all the way up to the smallest vessels. These vessels are so narrow that the flow rate will be reduced to roughly 1 inch (3 centimeters) per second. When the blood pressure is elevated on a long-term basis, the sensitive vascular walls will be threatened with irreparable damage—they simply cannot hold up under this constant strain.

When the Cause of High Blood Pressure Is Unknown

In 95 percent of all cases of high blood pressure, the doctors have no answers. An examination of the patient's organs and blood vessels usually will not point to an underlying illness as the cause. There may not even be the smallest clue to indicate that something is wrong. Yet the blood pressure is high. Specialists in hypertension describe this as "essential" or "primary" high blood pressure. It is believed that its causes are of a genetic nature.

Identifiable Causes of High Blood Pressure

In only 5 percent of all patients is it possible to determine an underlying cause for their condition. A frequent cause is arteriosclerosis, deposits on the inner walls of the blood vessels. This leads to a narrowing of the arteries and, as a result, a raise in blood pressure. What happens is comparable to a narrow point in a water hose, in which case the water pressure will increase. Less frequent causes of high blood pressure include illnesses of the kidneys, glands, or heart, as well as side effects of medications.

Measuring Blood Pressure

There are two readings that are obtained when your blood pressure is taken: the systolic and diastolic values. When the heart muscle contracts, it pumps blood from the left heart ventricle into the arteries, and a pressure wave runs through the vascular system. It can be felt in various places of the body as the pulse—at the neck or wrist, for example. If the blood pressure is measured at that moment, this will indicate the higher (systolic) value. The lower (diastolic) value measures the point at which the heart relaxes again. The heart ventricle extends, and the pressure in the vascular system drops temporarily until the heart pumps new blood again into the blood vessels.

MmHg stands for millimeters in mercury. This dates back to the days when blood pressure was measured by devices in which the mercury column was raised by pressure, and the change in height indicated the blood pressure values in millimeters.

Reference Values for Blood Pressure

The World Health Organization (WHO) divides the blood pressure scale into the following values:

Blood Pressure	Lower Value	Upper Value
High blood pressure	Above 95 mmHg	Above 160 mmHg
Borderline	Between 90 and 95 mmHg	Between 140 and 160 mmHg
Normal values	Up to 90 mmHg	Up to 140 mmHg

Symptoms and Consequences of High Blood Pressure

Only rarely does high blood pressure cause any noticeable symptoms, such as headaches or heart palpitations. But it is extremely harmful even without these symptoms. It causes eye damage as well as impairments in the functioning of the kidneys, which further elevate the blood pressure. High blood pressure also promotes the formation of arteriosclerosis, and this often ends up in a vicious cycle: The arteriosclerosis elevates the blood pressure, which in turn worsens the arteriosclerosis and leads to a further increase in blood pressure.

Modern devices for measuring blood pressure have highly sensitive sensors that are capable of registering precisely the moment of highest and lowest blood pressure and measuring it at that point.

Evening Primrose Oil for High Blood Pressure

Normally the blood is thin and runs smoothly through the blood vessels. Various hormones provide a balanced relationship between coagulation-promoting and coagulation-impeding substances. This equilibrium shifts only in an emergency. For instance, when there is a bleeding wound due to an injury, the blood will coagulate and the bleeding is stopped—blood platelets clump together and thus form a reliable closure to the wound. This is vital, because we might otherwise bleed to death from even a small wound. But when an undesirable shift of this equilibrium takes place within the vessels between the coagulation-promoting and coagulation-impeding substances so that there is an increased tendency for the blood to coagulate, the blood platelets will clump together and a thrombus will form; this is a dangerous blood clot that may occlude the vessels and thereby interrupt the flow of blood.

Prostaglandin E1, which is formed from the gamma-linolenic acid contained in evening primrose, for example, suppresses the clumping of the blood platelets. It helps to prevent the formation of blood clots and thus counteracts an elevation in blood pressure. You should therefore prepare as many foods as possible with evening primrose oil or from time to time go on a treatment plan with the oil. The recipes, beginning on page 82, are offered as a natural and effective method of prevention.

Hyperactivity in Children

If a child frequently has difficulty concentrating, gets carried away with the merest stimulation, and falls into crying fits after minor disappointments, a more serious condition may be at the root of this behavior: hyperactivity, also called attention deficit disorder or hyperkinesis. Some pediatricians believe that this may be the most common psychiatric disorder in children. Approximately 3 to 5 percent of all children suffer from it, and it occurs almost exclusively in boys.

Causes of Hyperactivity

Medical science has still not been able to detect the exact causes of hyperactivity. However, there are increasing indications that there may be several trigger mechanisms at work and possibly also in combination:

❦ Chronic illnesses that do not affect parts of the brain, such as impairments in the functions of the heart, lungs, and kidneys, as well as diabetes mellitus. There is also some discussion that hyperactivity may be caused by side effects stemming from medications that have been prescribed for these illnesses.

❦ Psychological problems developing from the child not feeling accepted by his or her environment and suffering from a lack of attention.

❦ Changes in the cerebral function, which can occur after meningitis, accompanying symptoms of a brain tumor, or due to a lack of oxygen suffered during birth.

Caution: The symptoms characteristic of hyperkinesis may show up temporarily during various phases in a child's development. They should be of concern only if they are present without interruption for a period of at least one year. Even then the child should always be diagnosed by an expert, such as a child psychiatrist.

Not every very lively child is automatically hyperactive. It is essential for children, in exploring their environment, to be active and to make use of their natural curiosity. But when children are totally uncontrollable and quickly lose interest in an activity, these may be indications of hyperactivity.

Important: If the diagnosis of hyperkinesis is confirmed, scolding and harsh discipline are definitely not the solution. This only serves to put the child under additional pressure and may actually worsen the condition.

The Feingold Diet with Evening Primrose Oil

According to studies gathered by the Hyperactive Children Support Group, a community agency established in Great Britain, children with hyperkinesis also display a deficiency in essential fatty acids as well as a heightened sensitivity to preservatives and artificial color and flavor additives. This is why a combination of evening primrose oil in combination with the Feingold diet is a recommended treatment.

This diet, named after Ben Feingold, M.D., a physician at the Kaiser Foundation Hospital in San Francisco, stresses natural nutrition. The diet includes, for example, a cereal of rolled oats with milk and untreated fruit. It is important that the grain products provide an ample supply of vitamins from the B-complex group and the fruit a sufficient supply of vitamin C.

The following evening primrose oil applications have also been used successfully as a supplement, which should be taken at breakfast time and with dinner.

Children from Two to Five Years Old

Massage the contents of two 500 mg capsules of evening primrose oil twice a day into the skin of your child's lower arm. If a sufficient sup-

Children naturally have a need to be physically active, which should be encouraged and carefully distinguished from hyperactivity.

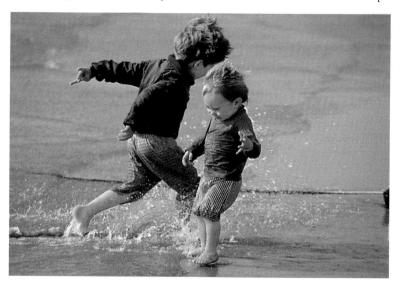

ply of vitamins cannot be obtained from food alone, you should give your child twice a day the following supplements in tablet form: 250 mg vitamin C, 15 mg pantothenic acid, and 50 mg vitamin B6. For children between two and five years of age, the evening primrose oil should be rubbed into the skin, because the absorption of the oil through the intestinal system may still be insufficient during the first few years of life. It can, however, easily penetrate through the skin and from there be absorbed completely into the body.

Children from Six to Seven Years Old

Give your child twice a day three 500 mg capsules of evening primrose oil, or rub the content of the capsules into the child's skin. If a sufficient supply of vitamins is not obtained through food, give your child twice a day these supplements in tablet form: 375 mg vitamin C, 22.5 mg pantothenic acid, and 75 mg vitamin B6.

Children from Seven Years Old and Up

Supplement the Feingold diet twice a day with four 500 mg capsules of evening primrose oil. Should there still be an insufficient vitamin supply through food, give your child twice a day in tablet form these supplements: 500 mg vitamin C, 30 mg pantothenic acid, and 100 mg vitamin B6. If no significant improvement is seen in a while, the evening primrose oil dosage can be increased to six capsules twice a day.

Helpful Hint: You can puncture the capsules with a needle and squeeze out the oil. Recipes for dishes prepared with evening primrose oil are in the recipe section, starting on page 82.

Menopausal Problems

According to statistics, the cessation of regular menstrual cycles, or menopause, nowadays starts in women between forty-nine and fifty-three years of age. The ovaries gradually cease to function, and the hormone levels change. The first indications of this change in the body—fatigue, nervousness, and headaches—can already be felt during what is known as perimenopause, the time prior to the last period.

Evening primrose oil is very easily digested, even among children. No side effects, with the exception of an occasionally soft stool, have been observed so far. If your child has trouble swallowing the capsules, you can puncture them and add the oil to tea, juice, or mineral water.

What Is the Source of the Problems?

The cause for menopausal problems lies first of all in the reduction of the estrogen level in the blood. The autonomic nervous system is out of balance, and the sympathetic nervous system reigns. The latter has a very stimulating effect and causes the body to become more active. Breathing and the heartbeat are accelerated, the blood pressure goes up, and the bronchial tubes and the coronary vessels become dilated. There is also a functional derailment within the brain: The center for the regulation of the body temperature located there will suddenly drive up the body temperature, resulting in hot flashes. And the hormone deficiency will cause a reduction in the release of the substances serotonin and noradrenalin within the brain. This results in an impairment of the normal dream state and of the deep stages of sleep.

Evening Primrose Oil for Menopausal Problems

Whether evening primrose oil can alleviate menopausal problems has still not been shown scientifically. However, some women state that taking evening primrose oil regularly in conjunction with melatonin and B-complex vitamins has improved their menopausal problems in a significant and lasting manner. Evening primrose oil can also be used in the form of a tea or as a bath oil.

Sleep may be interrupted during menopause. Also, all of a sudden, it may fail to provide the usual refreshment or relaxation. Instead, women often wake up in the morning already feeling fatigued and worn out.

Test with Evening Primrose Oil

At the Hospital for Obstetrics and Gynecology at Keele University in Stoke on Trent, Great Britain, twenty-eight women with menopausal problems were given a 500 mg capsule of evening primrose oil and 10 mg of vitamin E twice a day over a duration of six months. The women had to keep a diary over the span of the study to record the type and the severity of their problems. An evaluation of their diaries later showed that all of them recorded a significant reduction in nightly hot flashes.

Tea

Saint-John's-wort is effective in the treatment of depressive moods during menopause. It should be prepared as described on page 64 under "Premenstrual Syndrome (PMS)." At the beginning of this tea therapy, the dosage should be 2 cups per day. If the symptoms improve, this dosage can be reduced to 1 cup a day.

Bathing

Bath additives made from hay flowers have generally proven to be effective in the treatment of menopausal problems. Pour a little more than 1 gallon (5 liters) of water over 400 grams of hay flowers, and bring to a gradual boil. Simmer for 15 minutes on low heat, and then strain. Add this to the bathwater. The soothing effect is heightened with the addition of evening primrose oil. Stir 25 drops of oil into 1 cup of heavy cream, and add this to the bathwater. Be careful to keep the water temperature below 97°F (36°C), because evening primrose oil is very sensitive to heat.

Menstrual Disorders

A woman who never experienced a problem before may suddenly suffer from severe pain prior to or during her menstrual period. The bleeding will be much heavier than normal, and there will be back pain and possibly problems with bowel movements. Intercourse will be unexpectedly painful after her period. These may all be symptoms of endometriosis—next to a fibroid, the second most frequent benign abdominal disease for women. Approximately every tenth woman will have endometriosis at some point in her life.

What Is the Cause of Endometriosis?

Endometriosis is caused by cells that have separated from the lining of the uterus, the endometrium, and begin to move around. Why this happens is still largely unknown. One scientific explanation is as follows: During a normal period, there will usually be some cells from

Saint-John's-wort contains substances that are effective in the treatment of depressive moods and their physical manifestations. It can be taken in the form of juice, a tea, or an herbal tablet, and may be combined with evening primrose oil.

If the diagnosis is endometriosis, there is no cause for concern. This condition is almost always benign. However, you should still make an appointment with your gynecologist if you experience sudden pain during a period that you have never had before. This also holds true for any other problems that may occur in connection with your menstruation.

the lining of the uterus that are expelled along with blood. However, some of these cells will travel up the fallopian tube instead, reaching the pelvic cavity. They will settle in the ovaries, the muscles, the intestines, and the bladder, where they will attach themselves and multiply. They swell up there during menstruation. This puts pressure on the surrounding organs and therefore creates pain. If the endometrial cells settle on the ovaries, this may also cause adhesions and prevent ovulation—in fact, roughly 15 percent of all infertile women suffer from endometriosis.

Evening Primrose Oil in Relieving Endometriosis

Conventional medicine uses several treatment methods for endometriosis, such as gestagen preparations, medications with progesterone, as well as the possibility of a laparoscopy if treatment with medication has been unsuccessful.

But the pain related to endometriosis can be relieved with a much gentler method. A daily dosage of 1,500 mg of evening primrose oil in capsule form or 10 drops of pure oil three times a day, in combination with 800 mg of vitamin E and 2,000 mg of vitamin C, has proven to be effective.

Migraine

During migraine attacks, there will suddenly be an excess of messenger substances in the brain, which causes an inflammatory reaction in the brain vessels. This may lead to severe headaches on one side of the head, along with nausea and neurological impairments, such as zigzag lines and flickering shapes appearing in the line of vision.

Evening Primrose Oil Reduces the Pain

The exact effect of a therapy with evening primrose oil for migraine attacks has yet to be explained scientifically. However, in individual cases, beneficial results have been obtained. Certain patient reports

A serious case of endometriosis with enlarged growths causing severe pain can be treated surgically. However, surgery will usually be considered only as a last resort after all other therapies have failed.

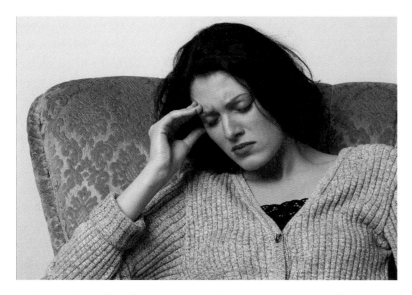

indicate that, after the ingestion of evening primrose oil, the time periods in between attacks grew longer and the pain became more tolerable.

The reduction in pain intensity, in particular, could be due to the affective mechanism of prostaglandin E1, which has been produced in the body with the help of the evening primrose oil. Prostaglandin E1 has been shown to have an anti-inflammatory effect, which might explain the lessening of the migraine pain.

Multiple Sclerosis

Multiple sclerosis is among the most frequent diseases of the central nervous system. But so far research has been unable to fully explain the causes of this illness. What is known is that, during its course, the immune system reacts to its own body tissue and progressively damages the nerves to such a degree that their function is reduced or even comes to a complete standstill. Patients will suffer from extensive paralysis, attacks of dizziness, and impairments in vision, speech, coordination, and the sensory system. It is typical for the disease to flare up during acute phases and to get progressively worse.

It is believed that a genetic predisposition, along with viruses and a diminished capacity of the body to metabolize fatty acids, plays a role in the cause of multiple sclerosis.

Delaying the Progress of the Disease

Several studies have shown that, by also taking evening primrose oil, the effectiveness of certain medications that slow down the progression of the illness and prolong the time intervals between acute phases may be increased.

Neurodermatitis

Neurodermatitus is a chronic allergic disorder of the skin. In many cases, the condition starts during the first few years of life. It was formerly believed that this skin disorder would go away with the onset of puberty. However, it has been found that the majority of all children suffering from neurodermatitis will continue to have it as adults.

The symptoms of neurodermatitis are burning and itching skin, predominantly on the inside of the elbows, behind the knees, at the neck, and on the hands, and red rashes in addition to running sores scattered over large parts of the body. The itching is particularly pronounced during the night. People will scratch themselves in states of partial sleep to such a degree that they break the surface of the skin, allowing bacteria to enter the body and cause infections.

What Causes Neurodermatitis?

What exactly triggers this condition is still not fully clear, although genetic predisposition is believed to play a large part. But genetics alone are not responsible for the onset of neurodermatitis. It is only when other factors come into play that there will be an outbreak. Such factors include environmental influences, allergies, stress, unresolved emotional problems, or an improper diet that is lacking in vitamins and minerals.

How Evening Primrose Oil Helps

Several studies have shown that, in patients afflicted with neurodermatitis, the conversion of linoleic acid into gamma-linolenic acid may

What else you can do if your child has neurodermatitis:

❦ If possible, eliminate all dust-catching articles from your child's room, such as carpeting, upholstered furniture, open shelves, and stuffed toys.

❦ Do not bathe your child too often, and always add moisturizing bath oils to the water.

❦ Use soy products as a substitute for dairy products.

❦ Refrain from smoking, because secondary smoke interferes with your child's immune system.

Intensive Treatment with Evening Primrose Oil

❦ In the treatment of neurodermatitis, the following dosage is recommended: Start with a two-month, intensive daily therapy of three to six 500 mg capsules of evening primrose oil.

❦ Following this, the treatment can be reduced to a maintenance therapy of two capsules twice a day or even only one capsule twice daily.

be impaired. Gamma-linolenic acid is extremely important for healthy, smooth skin. If there is a deficiency, the composition of the skin oils changes and the protective barrier function of the skin is impaired. The skin dries out, allowing bacteria and other pollutants to penetrate more easily. If the deficiency in gamma-linolenic acid is balanced with the regular ingestion of evening primrose oil, the skin irritations and infections will diminish, the itching will lessen, and the skin will be able to regenerate itself.

Useful applications are found in the chapter "Beauty Care with Evening Primrose Oil," starting on page 70.

Scientific Studies Prove Its Effectiveness

❦ At the University of Turku, Finland, fourteen patients suffering from neurodermatitis were given capsules of evening primrose oil over a period of twelve weeks. At the end of the twelve weeks, the doctors observed a significant reduction in their infections.

❦ A study undertaken over a duration of one year with 609 patients at various clinics was able to confirm the effectiveness of evening primrose oil. The adults took up to twelve 500 mg capsules of evening primrose oil per day, and the children up to six of the capsules per day. During the first three months, the affected skin surface was reduced from 37 percent down to 26 percent of the entire body surface. During the following nine months, this was further reduced down to 19 percent. During the first three months of the study, 43

Child psychologists have observed that the parents of children with neurodermatitis often make the mistake of doing too much for their children. Their excessive care will often contribute to making their children overly dependent. Instead, these children need to learn to cope with their condition and to take responsibility for their own treatment.

percent of the patients under observation suffered an acute phase of eczema; during the last three months, that number was reduced to only 16 percent. In every second patient, the symptoms improved to such a degree that no further medication became necessary.

Guidelines for Alleviating Neurodermatitis

Along with taking evening primrose oil, you should observe the following guidelines in order to alleviate the discomfort:

❧ When cleaning your home, avoid the whirling of dust when sweeping, for example, and use damp cloths instead.

❧ If possible, replace a feather or horsehair mattress with a mattress made from an artificial fiber material.

❧ Refrain from keeping pets in your home.

❧ Do not carry out any renovation work inside your home that requires applying paints, lacquers, thinners, or wood preservatives.

❧ Never wear wool or silk clothing; wear clothing made of pure cotton or a high-grade artificial fiber instead.

❧ Do not use aggressive detergents or laundry softeners.

❧ Do not bathe or shower excessively. Cleanse the skin only with water or with a mild, moisturizing bath or shower gel.

❧ Taking a shower is better than bathing. But never shower with hot water (it should be below 89°F, or 32°C), and don't stay in the shower longer than 5 to 10 minutes.

❧ Avoid the irritation of massaging brushes or rough sponges.

❧ Take baths with bath oils, and apply a moisturizing cream to your skin afterward. Don't forget your feet.

❧ To avoid contaminating your moisturizing-cream jar, remove the cream with a spatula or a spoon.

❧ When drying off, blot your skin rather than rubbing it dry.

Tips for people with symptoms of neuro-dermatitis:

❧ Always use gloves for housework.

❧ The chlorinated water in pools is often not tolerated. If it cannot be avoided, take care to rinse the skin well and to use a moisturizer.

❧ Avoid clothing made of wool or inferior artificial fibers, because they can irritate the skin, and look instead for clothing made from cotton.

Relieve the Itching with Evening Primrose Oil

You can support the intensive internal therapy with the topical application of salves, creams, or lotions containing evening primrose oil (from the health food store or the drugstore) that will help to regenerate the protective layer of the skin and nourish it. In addition, by gently applying pure evening primrose oil to the afflicted areas of the skin, you can relieve the agonizing itching. Even small amounts have a soothing effect.

Overweight

According to the American Medical Association, more than half of the adults in the United States are overweight or obese. Obesity can be defined as a 20 percent excess of body fat over one's ideal weight. The main cause of being overweight or obese is improper dietary habits. Lack of exercise ranks in second place. Many people spend hours in front of the television every night. On weekends, they also tend to be lazy. If they don't spend the weekend sitting around at home, they are generally sitting in a car on their way to see friends or relatives, and when they arrive at their destinations they usually spend some more time sitting down engaged in social conversation.

Health Consequences from Being Overweight

Diseases caused by improper nutrition include heart and coronary diseases, diabetes mellitus, stomach and colon cancer, kidney diseases, rheumatic disorders, and obesity. Obesity in turn is associated with higher rates of diabetes and diseases of the circulatory system and the kidneys. Obesity can also complicate existing illnesses, such as arthritis. Moreover, it is estimated that nearly every second illness ending in death is due to improper nutrition and being overweight.

Although nutrition experts recommend that no more than 25 percent of all calories be obtained from fat, the average fat consumption consists of about 40 percent of all calories consumed. And more than half of these are normally derived from animal fats, which means predominantly from saturated fats.

Ideal Weight Tables

What follow are sample "ideal" weights. (The weights are in pounds at ages twenty-five through fifty-nine and are based on the lowest mortality.)

Height	Small Frame	Medium Frame	Large Frame
Men			
5 ft. 4 in.	132–138	135–145	142–156
5 ft. 6 in.	136–142	139–151	146–164
5 ft. 8 in.	140–148	145–157	152–172
5 ft. 10 in.	144–154	151–163	158–180
6 ft.	149–160	157–170	164–188
6 ft. 2 in.	155–168	164–178	172–197
6 ft. 4 in.	162–176	171–187	181–207
Women			
5 ft.	104–115	113–126	122–137
5 ft. 2 in.	108–121	118–132	128–143
5 ft. 4 in.	114–127	124–138	134–151
5 ft. 6 in.	120–133	130–144	140–159
5 ft. 8 in.	126–139	136–150	146–167
5 ft. 10	132–145	142–156	152–173
6 ft.	138–151	148–162	158–179

> The pounds that are lost during a diet are often gained back just as quickly a short time later. The cause for this is the body's natural propensity to redouble its efforts in the storing of fat after "lean times"—that is, after a temporary withdrawal from food—in order to be better prepared for the next "starvation period."

How to Succeed on a Diet

There are numerous diets being advertised for weight reduction, most of which do not actually contribute to a sensible weight loss. The crash diets, in particular, will produce a sustained level of success in only the rarest of cases. In the opinion of experienced nutritionists, a long-term weight reduction program and the subsequent maintenance of a normal weight can be achieved only with a radical switch in eating habits. According to their recommendations, the daily calorie intake should be distributed as follows:

❧ 60 percent as carbohydrates

❧ 25 percent as fat, and half of that derived from plants

❧ 15 percent as protein

How the Pounds Will Melt Down

The way evening primrose oil contributes to weight reduction involves a still-not-fully-understood mechanism that is tied to the brown fat, which is a heat-producing tissue. When this mechanism is impaired and the communication between the center for the feeling of satisfaction located within the brain and the brown fat is interrupted, the brown fat cells will either not react at all or only very slowly to the command to burn up superfluous calories. These are then stored in the remaining fat cells of the body, creating a condition of being overweight.

This impaired mechanism can be restored with the help of evening primrose oil. It affects the mitochondrion, those power plants in the nucleus of the brown fat cells, in a manner that is still unexplained. These brown fat cells in turn power up the cellular metabolism, thus contributing to an increased burning of carbohydrates, which are available to the body in the form of energy. Excess fats are broken down, and the condition of being overweight is reduced or not even created in the first place.

The brown fat in the human body is found exclusively in the neck area and along the spine. It receives its name from its brownish coloring, which is due to a high concentration of mitochondrion. Brown fat, unlike body fat, does not produce energy during physical activity but merely serves to maintain the body temperature.

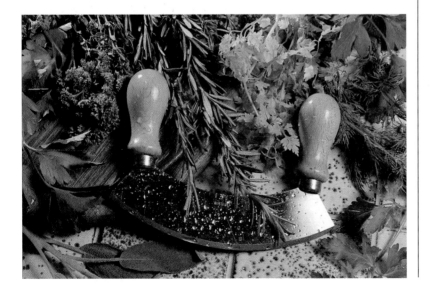

A person's ideal weight has to do with the percentage of body fat to total body weight. Roughly 18 percent for men and 21 percent for women are recommended.

Burning Calories through Exercise	
Activity	**Calories Burnt per Hour**
Jogging	600 cal.
Skiing	520 cal.
Climbing stairs	510 cal.
Swimming	430 cal.
Bicycling	330 cal.
Body exercises	300 cal.
Dancing	300 cal.
Very strenuous work	260 cal.
Cleaning windows	240 cal.
Walking	180 cal.
Strenuous work	180 cal.
Weeding	140 cal.
Light work	80 cal.

Research on the success of diets tells us the following:

❦ Only about one person out of 200 succeeds in maintaining the new weight for more than one year.

❦ Roughly 95 percent of all people having reduced their weight with the help of a diet will be heavier five years later than before the start of the diet.

❦ About 70 percent of all people who go on a diet end it prematurely.

Reduce Excess Weight with Evening Primrose Oil

Evening primrose oil can be used successfully to help reduce excess weight. This was discovered coincidentally over the course of research at Bootham Park Hospital in York, Great Britain, that was conducted in order to investigate the effects of gamma-linolenic acid on schizophrenics. The result was then confirmed by further studies.

Even if the precise connection between evening primrose oil and weight reduction is not yet fully clear, the results of these studies are still very encouraging. For instance, patients who were more than 10 percent overweight and took a daily dosage of eight 500 mg capsules of evening primrose oil as part of a research project at the University of Wales in Cardiff lost on an average 11 pounds (5 kilograms) of body weight over the course of six weeks. A therapy of evening primrose oil for people who are only slightly overweight will not show any effect, however. The weight loss occurred only in people who were more than 10 percent overweight.

Pregnancy Complications

Severe headaches, piercing pains in the abdomen, blurred vision, or cramps during the last weeks of pregnancy should never be neglected. If one or several of these symptoms occur, a doctor should be notified immediately—even at night—or the patient should be taken to a hospital. These symptoms may be the signs of a dangerous pre-eclampsia condition, which through complications could lead to a full-blown case of eclampsia and threaten the lives of both the expectant mother and the child.

What Is Pre-eclampsia?

During a pre-eclampsia phase, the blood pressure suddenly shoots up, increased protein is released through the urine and sometimes is also mixed with blood, and edemas may form throughout all the tissue of the body. The edemas are most likely the underlying cause of

Evening primrose oil is a harmless food supplement. Nevertheless, you should clarify with your doctor during your pregnancy whether or not he or she would recommend taking it and, if so, what the dosage should be.

Evening Primrose Oil Helps Prevent Pre-eclampsia

A study conducted at the School of Public Health and Tropical Medicine at Tulane University in New Orleans has shown that evening primrose oil can help to prevent the dangerous incidence of pre-eclampsia.

In the controlled double-blind study, one group of pregnant women received capsules with a mixture of evening primrose oil, fish oil, and magnesium oxide and another group was given only placebos. In those women who had been treated with the evening primrose oil mixture, there was not a single case of pre-eclampsia; in the test group receiving only placebos, there were three cases.

Recipes for meals with evening primrose oil with which you can maintain a healthy diet during pregnancy begin on page 82.

the severe headaches, as the accumulation of the liquid presses on the sensitive nerves in the head.

What Happens with Eclampsia?

Roughly half of all eclempsia cases, which may develop from the preliminary stage of pre-eclampsia, occur during the last weeks of pregnancy, and of these cases about a third take place during labor and delivery. If the pregnant woman is not treated immediately, she may fall into a coma or die instantly. The same may happen to the baby if it has not yet been delivered.

First Aid in Cases of Eclampsia

In the treatment of eclampsia, it is vital that the patient be taken to a hospital right away. Once there, she will be put on oxygen and be given anticonvulsive medications. In order to save the mother and the child, a cesarean will have to be performed without delay. Once the baby has been delivered, the symptoms, strangely enough, will disappear almost instantaneously.

Premenstrual Syndrome (PMS)

Between 50 to 70 percent of all women suffer from premenstrual syndrome during the days prior to their menstrual periods. The symptoms of PMS, which differ widely from woman to woman and cease with the start of the menstrual cycle, include swelling in the breasts or in the extremities, headaches, fatigue, attacks of ravenous hunger, depression, irritability, anxiety, lack of appetite, problems with concentration, back pain, sleep disorders, a bloated feeling, constipation, weight gain due to water retention in the body tissues, cramping in the stomach and the abdomen, loss of libido, and acne. The symptoms can start as many as fourteen days prior to the onset of the menstrual cycle, and they reach their climax between the fifth and second day prior to the period.

Women suffering from PMS produce an excessive amount of the hormone prolactin. They also suffer from a simultaneous deficiency in prostaglandin E1, which could stop this overproduction and regulate it. When evening primrose oil is ingested, the body converts it into prostaglandin E1, and the level of prolactin is balanced out again.

Evening Primrose Oil Is Found to Improve PMS

❦ The exact causes of PMS are as yet unknown, but doctors at the University of Otago in Dunedin, New Zealand, made an interesting observation: Probably due to hormonal changes, the blood in women suffering from PMS became increasingly thicker during the third week of the menstrual cycle. When these women ingested evening primrose oil, the blood became thinner again and the PMS symptoms lessened.

❦ Significant improvement in cases of PMS after the administration of evening primrose oil was also observed in a study involving sixty-five women conducted by Dr. Michael Brush at St. Thomas Hospital in London: In 61 percent of the women treated, the PMS problems disappeared entirely, and a partial improvement was seen in 23 percent of the women. Only 15 percent of the women stated that they felt no improvement. The evening primrose oil was administered in capsule form; the participants took two 500 mg capsules twice a day following a meal.

Prostaglandin E1 dilates the blood vessels and also affects the smooth consistency of the blood. This improves the blood circulation throughout the entire body.

Forms of Treatment with Evening Primrose Oil

There are two ways that evening primrose oil can be used to help-prevent PMS:

❦ Evening primrose oil can be taken in the form of capsules, which are available under several labels at drugstores and as a nutritive supplement at health food stores. The dosage varies from individual to individual, and may range from two to three or more capsules twice a day. It is best to start out with a lower dosage and to increase it gradually if there has been no improvement until an individual dosage has been established.

❦ Evening primrose oil can also be ingested as a pure oil. It is recommended to use a small amount daily during the days of the menstrual cycle when there are no symptoms—for example, 5 drops

In cases of PMS, plenty of physical exercise and sports in the open air support therapy with evening primrose oil. You should also try to avoid as much stress as possible during the critical days. If there is still no improvement despite all efforts, and if you are on birth control pills, try switching the medication. The symptoms may disappear altogether a short time later.

three times a day at mealtime—and then to increase this dosage at the onset of symptoms.

Evening Primrose Oil for PMS Depression

The plant dyes quercitrin and quercetin contained in Saint-John's-wort activate the neurotransmitter serotonin, which is capable of arousing feelings of happiness, so they help in this manner to control depressive moods. Tea made from Saint-John's-wort together with evening primrose oil is particularly suitable in the treatment of PMS when symptoms include irritability, nervousness, fearfulness, and depression.

Pour 1 cup of cold water over 1 heaping tablespoon of Saint-John's-wort, and heat this tea until boiling. Strain after 5 minutes. Let the tea cool to body temperature, and then add 5 to 10 drops of evening primrose oil mixed with 1 teaspoon of cold milk. You should test the individual dosage until you notice an improvement. In lighter cases, 1 cup daily may be enough to alleviate the symptoms during the critical days. However, it may also be possible that the daily dosage will have to be increased to 2 or 3 cups per day.

Fresh herbs—the potassium contained in them acts as an anticonvulsant in the presence of menstrual cramps. They also make it possible to use less salt in cooking.

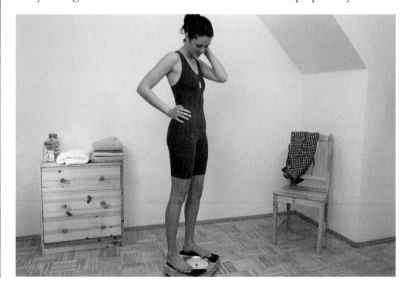

Dietary Guidelines for Premenstrual Syndrome

🐾 Your daily meal plan should include easily digestible nutrients that are rich in vitamins. Watch for a sufficient intake of vitamin B6, in order to support the conversion of gamma-linolenic acid to dihomo-gamma-linolenic acid.

🐾 Increase your intake of protein, because the protein ingested with your food reduces the outflow of liquids into the tissues, which is often the cause for the breasts and extremities feeling swollen. The protein can be obtained from milk and dairy products.

🐾 Make sure you get enough magnesium. Magnesium is found especially in wheat germ, wheat bran, millet, lentils, peas, soybeans, barley, nuts, corn, dairy products, rolled oats, and brewer's yeast.

🐾 Try to replace meat with fish. Fish contains omega-3 fatty acids, which also stimulate the prostaglandin metabolism and are capable of reducing PMS symptoms.

🐾 Try to do without salt, if possible, in order to counteract the retention of fluids in the tissues. At the same time, include foods such as potatoes and rice, which also help to dehydrate.

Rheumatic Disorders

The term "rheumatism" does not refer to one single, independent disease, but is an umbrella designation for nearly 400 different disorders. Common to all of them is severe pain in the muscles, joints, or fibrous tissue, and mobility may be significantly impaired as well.

What Causes Rheumatism?

According to new discoveries in medicine, rheumatic diseases are a type of auto-immune disease in which the immune system has gone awry and attacks the body. This leads to inflammations in the joints (rheumatoid arthritis), because the body's own defense mechanisms attack the lining of the joints and gradually destroy their sensitive tissues. An excess amount of prostaglandin E2, formed from arachi-

The first symptoms in all rheumatic diseases are very similar: aching joints or muscles as soon as one tries to move, such as after getting up in the morning. In the beginning phase, these symptoms will disappear on their own after the first few minutes and only return the next morning. But in time they will intensify and progressively worsen.

The body receives additional arachidonic acid through the intake of animal protein from foods such as meat, meat products, and eggs, and, with a normal diet, approximately ten times the amount needed per day is supplied. The excess supply causes an increased production of prostaglandin E2, bringing about a disruption in the balance between prostaglandin E1 and E2.

donic acid in the body, is largely responsible for the symptoms of inflammation. There is also a simultaneous deficiency in prostaglandin E1, which normally has an anti-inflammatory effect.

Prostaglandin E1 for Rheumatic Pain

Prostaglandin E1 has yet another positive effect on all rheumatic diseases:

❦ T-lymphocytes, the smallest white blood cells formed by the bone marrow, play an important part in all inflammations of the joints. Prostaglandin E1 can curb the excessive activity of these immune cells.

❦ The tissue damage that occurs in the joints of patients suffering from advanced rheumatic diseases is caused by certain enzymes that are released during an inflammatory phase from the lyosomes, minute parts of each cell. Prostaglandin E1 is capable of stopping the release of these enzymes and can therefore act effectively against the feared tissue damage.

❦ In addition to prostaglandin E2, the arachidonic acid produces inflammation-promoting leukotriene, which are also part of the rheumatic disorder. Doctors at Royal North Shore Hospital at the

The Effect of Evening Primrose Oil on Rheumatism

❦ Rheumatism medications, such as the non-steroidal antirheumatica, block the conversion of arachidonic acid into the inflammation-promoting prostaglandin E2.

❦ Evening primrose oil has a similar effect. When it is ingested, the body will increase the production of prostaglandin E1 from gamma-linolenic acid. An increase in the level of the anti-inflammatory prostaglandin E1 automatically causes a reduction in the inflammation-promoting prostaglandin E2 level by suppressing the production of prostanglandin E2 from the arachidonic acid.

Arachidonic Acid Content in Foods

Foods (per 3.5 oz., or 100 g, of edible portion)	Arachidonic Acid (in mg)
Milk and Dairy Products	
Cow's milk (3.5 % fat)	4
Cow's milk (1.5 % fat)	2
Whey	0
Curd cheese (similar to cottage cheese) (20% fat)	5
Curd cheese (low-fat)	0
Camembert	34
Eggs	
Egg (whole egg)	70
Egg yolk	297
Fats and Oils	
Pork lard	1,700
Diet margarine	0
Wheat germ oil	0
Meat and Meat Products	
Pork liver	870
Liverwurst	230
Pork meat (muscle)	120
Beef meat (muscle)	70
Chicken	112
Veal	53
Vegetables, potatoes, nuts	0
Soy products	0
Fruit	0

Source: Adam, O.: Arachidonsäuregehalt in ausgewählten Lebensmitteln (Arachidonic Acid Content in Selected Foods). In: Aktuelle Ernährungsmedizin 20 (1995), p. 183.

The body requires arachidonic acid in order to maintain elasticity in the cells. But it is also the basic substance for the production of prostaglandin E2. Normally the body only releases as much acid as is needed. However, frequently an excess will be produced through the intake of too much animal protein.

Rheumatic disorders include the following:

❦ **Osteoarthritis (degeneration of the joints)**

❦ **Rheumatoid arthritis (inflammation of the joints)**

❦ **Polyarthritis (arthritis involving two or more joints)**

❦ **Gout (inflammation of the joints, with deposits of urates in and around the joints and excessive uric acid in the blood)**

❦ **Rheumatic fever (fever, inflammation, pain, swelling in and around the joints)**

University of Sidney, Australia, were able to prove that the ingestion of evening primrose oil prevents the production of leukotriene.

Correct Dosage Is Important

A therapy with evening primrose oil requires patience. As a rule, an improvement will only be noticeable after three months. In his book *Evening Primrose Oil,* Richard A. Passwater has the following to say about the treatment of rheumatic disorders with evening primrose oil: "In some patients an improvement could be observed when a daily dosage of 3 or 4 grams of evening primrose oil was administered. This means every morning and every evening three or four 500 mg capsules of evening primrose oil." In order to avoid an excess of arachidonic acid especially in the bodies of patients with rheumatic diseases, not more than 80 milligrams should be ingested through the daily intake of food. See the table on page 67 for the arachidonic acid content of various foods.

Massage the Pain Away

Rheumatic pain can be alleviated with a massage oil made from avocado, evening primrose, and tea tree oil. Add 30 drops each of evening primrose and tea tree oil to 100 ml of avocado oil. Massage the aching joint with this mixture twice a day.

Remedies for Rheumatic Disorders

❦ Maintain a balanced diet that is rich in vitamins and minerals and includes plenty of fresh fruit and vegetables. Reduce your consumption of meat, and try to do without animal fats.

❦ Lose weight, if necessary. Excess pounds put pressure on the joints and aggravate rheumatoid arthritis, in particular.

❦ Try to purify your body regularly. Especially in patients suffering from rheumatism, the tissues have absorbed numerous waste products. Plan to fast for a week. Drink ample amounts of purification teas made from birch, elder, dandelion, yarrow, or nettle.

❦ Take care that you get enough exercise in the open air, and walk daily for at least half an hour—even if it hurts at times.

❦ Avoid stress, and get a minimum of 8 hours of sleep at night. Also, include several brief rest periods during the day, during which you should try to relax both body and soul.

❦ Avoid activities that involve only one part of the body. Do not complete all housework in one stretch, but alternate with lighter work in between.

❦ Your bed and couches and chairs should not be too soft but instead should give you firm support, in order to minimize the weight load on your body.

❦ During acute phases of rheumatism, you can promote the regeneration of the body by giving it a rest. Lie down during these times as much as possible.

Schizophrenia

In actuality, schizophrenia does not correspond to the commonly accepted notion of a split personality or a split consciousness. It appears instead that those people who are afflicted suffer from a loss of contact with the environment and from delusions and hallucinations that are due to a biochemical dysfunction. The delusions range from paranoia or megalomania to obsessive jealousy or the delusional idea of being another person. During the hallucinatory phase, the patient may hear voices or see people who do not exist in reality. However, patients at Bootham Park Hospital in York, Great Britain, have shown a significant improvement when treated with evening primrose oil in combination with penicillin.

The cause of schizophrenia has still not been determined. Scientists hypothesize that each individual case represents an unfavorable combination of biographic, psychological, neurological, and genetic conditions.

Seasonal Affective Disorder (SAD)

In individual cases, people suffering from winter depression, or seasonal affective disorder (SAD), have reported a noticeable improvement in their condition when they took evening primrose oil together with vitamins from the B-complex group.

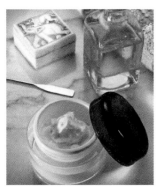

Cosmetics made from evening primrose oil can be easily prepared at home.

Problem skin as well as healthy skin can benefit from the effects of evening primrose oil, because it supports the natural functions of the skin and prevents premature wrinkling.

Beauty Care with Evening Primrose Oil

Skin Care

The skin is the body's largest organ. The skin plays an important role in the excretion of metabolic waste products by means of its oil and sweat glands. At the same time, it protects the body from pathogens from the environment, such as viruses or bacteria. To ensure the smooth functioning of the skin as an excretory organ and an environmental barrier, it needs to stay soft and supple and its metabolism must remain undisturbed. When the skin becomes rough and dry or wrinkled, it is a sign that it is suffering from a deficiency in vital substances. Evening primrose oil can prevent a deficiency in nutrients or even repair the damage if a deficiency has already occurred. In this manner, it contributes to skin that is well cared for, youthful, and free of wrinkles.

Face and Body Creams

Basic Day Cream

Ingredients: 40 g of a glyceryl stearate (a non-self-emulsifier), 80 g of sunflower oil, and 30 g of cocoa butter.

Preparation: You will need two pans. Heat the glyceryl stearate and the sunflower oil in one pan until they are mixed thoroughly. You must not let these ingredients get too hot, otherwise this could destroy their valuable oil substances. As soon as the mixture has cooled down to around 104°F (40°C), carefully add the cocoa butter, which you have melted in the second pan.

This basic cream will serve as a base for making additional creams with evening primrose oil and other skin-nourishing substances. Because evening primrose oil as well as certain other aromatic oils are very sensitive to heat, the other ingredients should be added only when the cream base has cooled to below 95°F (35°C). It would be best to add the evening primrose oil last, when you are barely able to still stir the mixture. The various ingredients for creams for specific skin types are listed below.

Basic Night Cream

Ingredients: 40 g of a glyceryl stearate (a non-self-emulsifier), 50 g of avocado oil, 30 g of sunflower oil, and 30 g of cocoa butter.

Preparation: The preparation follows the same basic procedure as described for the day cream. The glyceryl stearate, avocado oil, and sunflower oil are heated together. The cocoa butter should be added only after the mixture cools down to about 104°F (40°C).

The avocado oil, which is rich in vitamins, penetrates the skin easily and has a lubricating and moisturizing effect. It will, however, produce a slightly oily sheen on the skin, which is why it is omitted from the preparation of the day cream.

You can also prepare a night cream for your own skin type with the following individualized mixtures for day cream. But you will use the basic night cream as a base instead of the basic day cream.

Special Creams for Every Skin Type

Day Cream for Normal Skin

Ingredients: Add 15 drops each of aloe vera and jojoba oil, 20 drops of rose oil, and 10 drops of evening primrose oil to the basic day cream.

Day Cream for Dry Skin

Ingredients: Add 8 drops of geranium oil and 12 drops each of lavender and evening primrose oil to the basic day cream.

In extremely rare cases, every aromatic oil described here, including evening primrose oil, may cause an allergic reaction. You should therefore always make the following test prior to the first application: Apply 1 or 2 drops of the oil or the oil mixture to the inside of the elbow, which is one of the most sensitive places on the human body. If there is no reddening of the skin or no welts have formed, you haven't any cause for concern.

The skin creams with evening primrose oil for each specific skin type produce beautiful and clear skin.

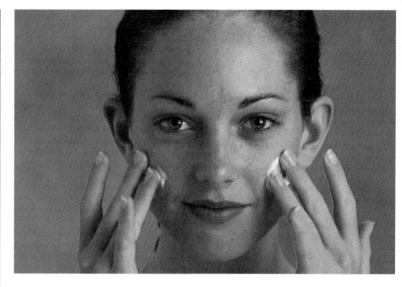

Day Cream for Oily Skin

Ingredients: Add 10 drops of bergamot oil, 6 drops each of lemon and sandalwood oil, and 8 drops of evening primrose oil to the basic day cream.

Day Cream for Aging Skin

Ingredients: Add 8 drops each of neroli and sandalwood oil, 6 drops of orange oil, and 15 drops of evening primrose oil to the basic day cream.

Day Cream for Chapped or Inflamed Skin

Ingredients: Add 10 drops of chamomile oil, 6 drops each of sage and rosewood oil, and 10 drops of evening primrose oil to the basic day cream.

Cream for Wrinkles around the Eyes ("Crow's-Feet")

Ingredients: Add 4 drops each of chamomile and lavender oil, 6 drops of sandalwood oil, and 8 drops of evening primrose oil to the basic day cream.

Tip: Apply the cream carefully, taking care not to get any of it into your eyes because it may cause irritations.

Evening primrose oil is absorbed easily into the skin. It doesn't leave an unpleasant oily film, is moisturizing, and renders the skin velvety-soft.

Cream for Varicose Veins and Split Veins

Ingredients: Add 4 drops each of juniper essence and yarrow oil, 6 drops each of cypress and lemon oil, and 10 drops of evening primrose oil to the basic day cream.

Cellulite Cream

Ingredients: Add 8 drops each of yarrow and grapefruit oil, 4 drops of juniper essence, 10 drops of orange oil, and 12 drops of evening primrose oil to the basic day cream.

Cottage Cheese Facial Mask to Regenerate the Skin

Ingredients: ¼ of an 8 oz. (250 g) carton of low-fat cottage cheese, 2 tablespoons water, 1 tablespoon honey, 2 drops each of geranium and chamomile oil, 3 drops each of rosewood and lavender oil, and 5 drops of evening primrose oil.

Preparation: Take a fourth of the contents of an 8 oz. (250 g) carton of low-fat cottage cheese, and add 2 tablespoons of lukewarm water and 1 teaspoon of honey. Mix well, and then add the oils.

Apply this mixture to your face, and leave it on for 10 to 15 minutes. Rinse with lukewarm water. If a residue remains on your skin, don't remove it with soap but just with plenty of clear water.

Watch for quality when you purchase ingredients for homemade cosmetics. Naturally pure and high-grade products are available at health food stores, herb shops, and some drugstores, as well as through special mail-order companies.

Facial Mask for Dry Skin

Ingredients: 1 egg yolk, ¼ of an 8 oz. (250 g) carton of low-fat cottage cheese, 5 drops of rose oil, 3 drops of chamomile oil, and 10 drops of evening primrose oil.

Preparation: First stir the egg yolk into the low-fat cottage cheese, followed by the various oils. Apply this mixture to the face, and leave it on for 20 minutes. Then rinse with plenty of lukewarm water.

Tip: This mask should be used once a week. Try taking a warm bath with some evening primrose oil added for relaxation (see page 78) while keeping the mask on your face.

Nourishing Body Oils

Cleansing Oil for the Skin

Ingredients: 100 g sunflower oil, 10 drops evening primrose oil, 10 g lecithin CM, and 3 drops lavender oil.
Preparation: Thoroughly mix all ingredients.

Basic Body Oil

Ingredients: 50 g jojoba oil and 50 g wheat germ oil.
Preparation: Mix the two oils together; this will give you a base for all the individualized formulas that follow. By adding other ingredients, you can then produce an oil that is especially suitable for your own type of skin.

Oil for Dry Skin

Ingredients: Add 8 drops of honey, 8 drops of sandalwood oil, and 12 drops each of chamomile and evening primrose oil to the basic body oil.

Oil for Oily Skin

Ingredients: Add 6 drops of geranium oil and 10 drops each of cedar, ylang-ylang, and evening primrose oil to the basic body oil.

Oil for Blemished Skin

Ingredients: Add 8 drops each of rockrose and lavender oil as well as 12 drops each of pearly everlasting and evening primrose oil to the basic body oil.

Oil for Wrinkled and Aging Skin

Ingredients: Add 6 drops of sage oil, 10 drops each of neroli and galbanum oil, and 15 drops of evening primrose oil to the basic body oil.

Evening Primrose Oil Balm for Dry Skin

Ingredients: 40 g each of wheat germ and jojoba oil, 10 drops each of orange and laurel oil, 6 drops clove oil, 4 drops rose oil, and 10 drops evening primrose oil.
Preparation: Thoroughly mix all oils together.

The cosmetic formulas shown here are very easy to prepare. If you still don't want to bother, health food stores and drugstores now offer a steadily increasing selection of cosmetic products containing evening primrose oil.

Nourishing and Regenerating Body Lotions

Basic Lotion

Ingredients: 40 g each of jojoba and avocado oil as well as 20 drops evening primrose oil.
Preparation: You can then add various other ingredients, depending on your skin type.

Lotion for Oily Skin and Plugged Pores

Ingredients: Add 8 drops each of lavender, bergamot, cedar wood, and juniper oil to the basic lotion.

Lotion for Inflamed and Overstressed Skin

Ingredients: Add 8 drops each of chamomile, rose, geranium, and neroli oil to the basic lotion.

Lotion for Dry Skin

Ingredients: Add 10 drops of geranium oil and 8 drops each of sandalwood, ylang-ylang, and patchouli oil to the basic lotion.

Healing Oils

Oil for Insect Bites

Ingredients: 5 drops each of tea tree, lavender, lemon balm, and mint oil as well as 10 drops of evening primrose oil.
Preparation: Thoroughly mix all oils together, and apply to the bite several times a day. This will alleviate itching, redness, and swelling of the skin due to bee, wasp, or mosquito bites.

Oil for First-Degree Burns

Ingredients: 20 drops each of lavender and evening primrose oil.
Preparation: Mix the two oils, and apply to the burnt skin. This will help to alleviate the pain, prevent blistering, and support the rapid regeneration of the burnt skin.

Evening primrose oil in combination with certain other aromatic oils can also be used to treat skin injuries and even skin diseases. Here is an oil formula for athlete's foot: 30 g each of jojoba and aloe vera oil, 10 drops each of myrrh, tea tree, and lavender oil, and 15 drops of evening primrose oil. Add the aromatic oils to the two basic oils, and apply five times daily to the areas of the foot affected with the fungus.

Oil for Sunburn

Ingredients: 30 g each of aloe vera and jojoba oil, 15 drops each of lavender and chamomile oil, and 20 drops of evening primrose oil.
Preparation: Thoroughly mix all oils together, and apply to the sunburnt areas several times a day.

Oil for Hemorrhoids

Ingredients: 10 drops each of myrrh and cypress oil, 8 drops yarrow oil, 12 drops evening primrose oil, and 50 g jojoba oil.
Preparation: Add all the aromatic oils, including the evening primrose oil, to the jojoba oil, and mix them together. Apply a few drops three times a day to the afflicted area around the anus.

Oil for Sore Muscles

Ingredients: 40 g each of jojoba and wheat germ oil, 10 drops each of rosemary and marjoram oil, and 15 drops each of geranium and evening primrose oil.
Preparation: Thoroughly mix all oils together, and use to massage the sore muscles several times a day.

Healing oils for minor skin infections:

❦ **50 g jojoba oil**

❦ **10 drops geranium oil**

❦ **5 drops rose oil**

❦ **5 drops lavender oil**

❦ **10 drops evening primrose oil**

Disinfecting Smaller Wounds with Evening Primrose Oil

Ingredients: 10 drops each of bergamot, lavender, and evening primrose oil as well as 8 drops each of eucalyptus and rose oil.
Preparation: Thoroughly mix the oils together. Minor skin injuries, such as tears or cuts, can be disinfected easily with this mixture by applying it directly to the wound. The evening primrose oil supports the healing of the wound, whereas the other essential oils have a disinfecting property.

You can also prepare a wound cream by taking 20 g of beeswax and heating it to approximately 104°F (40°C) and then stirring it into the oil mixture. When the mixture cools, it firms up and can easily be rubbed into the skin. The beeswax contains additional substances that effectively disinfect and heal wounds.

Evening Primrose Oil for Herpes

Ingredients: 8 drops each of eucalyptus, lemon balm, and bergamot oil as well as 10 drops of evening primrose oil.

Preparation: Thoroughly mix all oils together. The area of the skin afflicted with herpes should be cleaned with lavender oil prior to the application of the oil mixture. Apply a few drops of lavender oil on some cotton, and cleanse the skin well. You can then rub in the anti-herpes mixture. Apply five times daily.

Evening Primrose Oil for Acne

Ingredients: 8 drops each of geranium, sandalwood, lavender, and lemon oil as well as 10 drops each of calendula and evening primrose oil.

Preparation: Thoroughly mix the oils together. Acne is caused by an overproduction of the male hormone testosterone, which leads to an increased formation of sebum in the sebaceous glands. A simultaneous formation of keratin at the outlet of the glands prevents the discharge of sebum. The sebum sacks swell up until the sebum is finally discharged through tiny skin fissures surrounding the glandular outlet. This leads to infections that are seen as acne pustules on the surface of the skin. The evening primrose oil in this acne oil has a regenerative and healing effect, whereas the other essential substances disinfect the skin and open up the pores.

Bath Additives with Evening Primrose Oil

Baths with the addition of evening primrose oil will keep the skin healthy, support the skin metabolism, and help to prevent wrinkles. The water temperature should never exceed 96.8°F (36°C), because the active ingredients in the oil might otherwise be damaged. Evening primrose oil should not be added directly to the bathwater, as the drops would float on the surface of the water like drops of grease. There are a number of emulsifiers—such as milk, cream, buttermilk, and honey—that allow the oil to be distributed evenly into the water.

In order to effectively treat outbreaks of herpes, the oil mixture should be applied at the first sign of symptoms, such as a slight itching in the area around the mouth. The sooner it is applied, the more successful it will be in preventing an eruption of herpes blisters.

Relaxing massage oil for menstrual problems:

❧ 25 g each of jojoba and wheat germ oil

❧ 20 drops each of juniper, bergamot, sage, fennel, and jasmine oil

❧ 20 drops of evening primrose oil

The following basic formula with the addition of various oils will enable you to create relaxing bath oils that may even promote your circulation.

Basic Bath Oil

Ingredients: 1 cup of cream or 2 cups of milk or buttermilk, 2 tablespoons of honey, and 20 to 25 drops of evening primrose oil.
Preparation: First add the honey and then the evening primrose oil to the cream or milk. Stir the mixture, and add it to the bathwater.

Invigorating and Regenerating Bath Oil

Ingredients: Add 5 to 8 drops each of cedar wood, stone pine, white cedar, sage, juniper, mountain pine, cypress, ginger, cajeput, coriander, and jasmine oil to the basic bath oil.

Soothing and Relaxing Bath Oil

Ingredients: Add 5 to 8 drops each of rose, neroli, sandalwood, ylang-ylang, lavender, geranium, olibanum, and chamomile oil to the basic bath oil.

Care for the Lips

For instant relief from chapped lips in wintertime or to prevent chapped lips, you can puncture a capsule of evening primrose oil and apply the oil directly to the lips without adding any other ingredients.

Evening primrose oil provides excellent protection for the lips. Chapped and dry lips will soon be soft and smooth again.

Lip Balm

Ingredients: 20 g honey, 10 g beeswax, 15 g jojoba oil, 2 drops lavender oil, and 4 drops evening primrose oil.
Preparation: First mix the honey into the slightly heated beeswax. Then add the oils, and stir everything well. Apply this balm to your lips several times a day.

Lipstick

Ingredients: 10 g beeswax, 10 g wheat germ oil, 20 g coconut oil, 10 g honey, 1 drop peppermint oil, and 4 drops evening primrose oil.

Preparation: First melt the beeswax in a pan together with the wheat germ oil. Next, add the coconut oil followed by the honey. After the mixture cools to the point where it can hardly be stirred, add the peppermint and evening primrose oil. You can then fill two empty, well-cleaned lipstick containers with this healing mixture.

Hair Care

For every hair problem, there is just the right evening primrose oil preparation. Especially if the scalp is lacking in oil or in the case of a metabolic disorder—both of which may be the cause of hair loss— hair treatments with evening primrose oil may be of help. Hair loss can often be lessened, and the hair becomes soft and silky again.

Basic Oil Treatment

Preparation: Mix all the ingredients listed under the individualized formulas at room temperature, and massage this solution into your hair. Wrap a towel around your head, and leave this mixture on for 1½ to 2 hours; then wash it out with a mild shampoo. You should use this oil pack about once a week.

The various ingredients for the different hair types are listed below. These oil treatments are prepared and applied following the same instructions as for the basic oil treatment.

Oil Treatment for Split Ends or Damaged Hair

Ingredients: 40 g wheat germ oil, 10 g jojoba oil, 5 drops sandalwood oil, and 10 drops each of rose and evening primrose oil.

Oil Treatment for Dandruff

Ingredients: 40 g wheat germ oil, 10 g jojoba oil, 5 drops each of rosemary, lime, and eucalyptus oil, and 10 drops evening primrose oil.

Hair loss may have several causes, including hormonal imbalances, exhaustion, psychological factors such as stress, vitamin or mineral deficiencies, and metabolic disorders. A further cause may be an oil deficiency in the scalp. A treatment with evening primrose oil could help.

Oil Treatment for Oily Hair

Ingredients: 40 g almond oil, 10 g jojoba oil, 5 drops each of lime, bergamot, and rosemary oil, and 10 drops evening primrose oil.

Oil Treatment for Dry Hair

Ingredients: 40 g almond oil, 10 g jojoba oil, 5 drops each of chamomile, sandalwood, and lavender oil, and 10 drops evening primrose oil.

Oil Treatment for Hair Loss

Ingredients: 40 g wheat germ oil, 12 drops cedar oil, 8 drops tea tree oil, 5 drops juniper oil, and 10 drops evening primrose oil.

Our fingernails are a reflection of our state of health. A normal fingernail is slightly longer than wide and has a smooth surface with a light sheen. The skin underneath the nail should be rosy-pink.

Nail Care

Evening primrose oil also helps to maintain beautiful nails. The participants in two studies conducted in Great Britain took two 500 mg capsules of evening primrose oil three times a day, and their problems with brittle and split nails disappeared.

Nails will also become firm and hard again within a short period of time when evening primrose oil is massaged directly into them. Rub 1 drop of evening primrose oil once a day into each nail.

Care of Toenails and Fingernails with Evening Primrose Oil

Ingredients: 100 ml wheat germ or jojoba oil, 10 drops each of cypress and sandalwood oil, 5 drops lavender oil, and 15 drops evening primrose oil.

Preparation: Mix the ingredients, and transfer into a bowl. Soak your nails in the mixture for 15 minutes a day. Afterward, you can pour the oil into a small bottle that closes well and store it for the next use.

Foot Care

Basic Foot Bath

Ingredients: 1 cup of cream or 2 cups of milk or buttermilk, 2 table-spoons of honey, and 5 to 10 drops of evening primrose oil.

Preparation: Thoroughly mix all ingredients together, and use this mixture as a base for a soothing foot bath. The water temperature should not exceed 96.8°F (36°C).

Foot Bath for Tired Feet

Ingredients: Add 3 drops each of rosemary and lavender oil to the foot-bath base.

Foot Bath for Sweaty Feet

Ingredients: Add 2 drops each of cypress and tea tree oil as well as 3 drops of lemon grass oil to the foot-bath base.

Foot Bath for Swollen Feet

Ingredients: Add 3 drops each of juniper and lavender oil as well as 2 drops of peppermint oil to the foot-bath base.

Foot Bath for Aching Feet

Ingredients: Add 3 drops each of sage and bergamot oil as well as 2 drops of juniper oil to the foot-bath base.

Cream for Corns

Ingredients: 25 g beeswax, 10 g cocoa butter, 60 ml avocado oil, 10 drops each of lemon, myrrh, chamomile, and lavender oil, and 15 drops evening primrose oil.

Preparation: Place the beeswax, the cocoa butter, and the avocado oil in a glass, and immerse the glass into a tub of water at a temperature of approximately 158°F (70°C). As soon as the mixture has melted, stir it up so that it is blended evenly. When it has cooled down to about 104°F (40°C), add the oils.

This is what you will need for a deodorant oil to prevent foot odor: 50 g jojoba or wheat germ oil, 5 drops each of lavender and tea tree oil, and 8 drops evening primrose oil. Mix the jojoba or wheat germ oil with the aromatic oils. Massage this mixture into your feet when you get up in the morning. This foot-deodorant oil will effectively protect you from foot odor throughout the day.

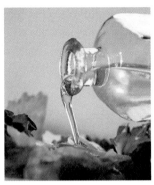

Evening primrose oil is also a cooking ingredient that is good for our health.

The addition of vitamin E assures the relatively long shelf life of evening primrose oil. Although the pure, freshly pressed oil from the seeds of evening primrose keeps for only a few weeks because it oxidizes rapidly, the protection that takes place through the addition of vitamin E delays the oxidation process significantly.

Cooking with Evening Primrose Oil

Evening primrose oil is a highly suitable ingredient in food preparation. In order to ensure the effectiveness of the oil components, though, one condition always has to be met: The foods that evening primrose oil is added to must not exceed a temperature of 95°F (35°C).

Because evening primrose oil combines easily with other vegetable oils, you can simply add it to the oil you normally use in the preparation of salads or other cold dishes. Evening primrose oil by itself has only a slight taste of its own, so, in adding it to other oils, you can hardly taste the difference.

As a rule of thumb, use 25 oz. (750 ml) of salad oil to 1 oz. (30 ml) of evening primrose oil. This dosage will automatically supply you in any salad dish with the valuable linoleic and gamma-linolenic acid from the evening primrose oil. Commercially available evening primrose oil usually keeps for one to one and a half years, so you needn't be concerned about early spoilage that might ruin the entire oil mixture.

Salads with Evening Primrose Oil

Tuna and Bean Salad

Ingredients: 1 can mushrooms (7 oz., or 200 g), 1 can tuna (5 to 6 oz., or 150 to 180 g), 1 can green beans (5 oz., or 150 g), 1 tablespoon each of parsley and basil, 4 tablespoons olive oil, 10 drops evening primrose oil, splash of lemon juice, salt, and pepper.

Preparation: Cut the mushrooms into slices, and place them, along with the tuna and the beans (both drained), in a salad bowl. Mince the fresh herbs, and mix them carefully with the olive and evening primrose oil and the lemon juice so that the tuna pieces don't fall apart. Season to taste with salt and pepper. The salad is best if you let it marinate for about 20 minutes, in order to allow the aroma to fully develop.

The quantities indicated in the recipes are for two people.

Bell Pepper Salad with Cider Vinegar

Ingredients: 2 each of red, green, and yellow bell peppers, 1 onion, 2 cloves garlic, 2 tablespoons cider vinegar, pepper, salt, 5 tablespoons olive oil, 10 drops evening primrose oil, and 50 black pitted olives.

Preparation: Cut the washed bell peppers in half, removing the seeds and the stems. Cut the peppers lengthwise into thin strips, and the onion into rings. Place the pepper strips into a salad bowl, and add the crushed garlic cloves. Toss the salad with the cider vinegar, pepper, salt, and the olive and evening primrose oil. Garnish with the onion rings and the olives. Place the salad in the refrigerator, and allow to chill for 30 minutes before serving.

Bell peppers contain a lot of vitamin B6, without which the body cannot convert the gamma-linolenic acid into dihomo-gamma-linolenic acid (the basic substance for prostaglandin E1).

Mushroom-Bean Salad with Watercress

Ingredients: 1 onion, 1.7 oz. (50 g) butter, 1 lb. (450 g) frozen green beans, 1 tablespoon tomato paste, 1 can mushrooms (7 oz., or 200 g), 1 bunch watercress, 2 garlic cloves, 4 tablespoons red wine vinegar, 5 tablespoons olive oil, 15 drops evening primrose oil, salt, and pepper.

Preparation: Finely chop the onion, and sauté in a pan until soft. Add the beans and the tomato paste, and let simmer for about 10 minutes. Rinse the mushrooms in a colander under warm water, cut into thin slices, and place them into a salad bowl along with the lukewarm beans and the other cooked ingredients. Put the trimmed watercress on top after washing and drying it. When the salad mixture has cooled sufficiently, add the crushed garlic cloves, the red wine vinegar, and the olive and evening primrose oil. Season to taste with salt and pepper, and mix well.

Mushrooms contain nicotine amide, which is necessary for the conversion of dihomo-gamma-linolenic acid into prostaglandin E1.

Greek Vegetable Salad

Ingredients: 2 bell peppers, 4 zucchinis, 2 eggplants, 5 large onions, 2 pepperonis, 1 cup chicken broth, 5.2 oz. (150 g) goat cheese, 20 drops evening primrose oil, 3 tablespoons olive oil, ½ bunch parsley, 4 tablespoons lemon juice, salt, pepper, and thyme.

Preparation: Wash the vegetables. Cut the bell peppers in half, removing the seeds. Slice the zucchinis, the eggplants, the onions, the pepperonis, and the peppers. Place the vegetables and the chicken broth into a pan with a high rim, and steam briefly. Strain, but reserve the broth. Cut the goat cheese into cubes. Mix the evening primrose oil into the olive oil. When the vegetables have cooled, add the goat cheese, the oil mixture, finely minced parsley, and the lemon juice. If the mixture appears too dry, add the remainder of the chicken broth. Season to taste with salt and pepper, and sprinkle with a little thyme.

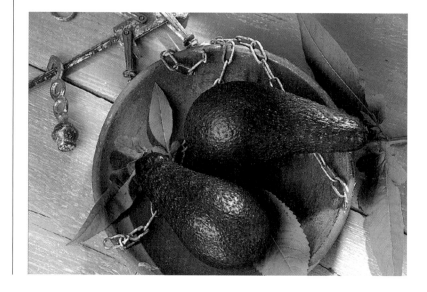

Avocados are ripe and fresh when their fruit pulp is just soft to the touch but cannot be pushed in too deeply. They will keep for three to four days when stored in a cool place.

Snacks

Evening primrose oil can also be used to supplement cold snacks in between meals—and you will be doing something for your health at the same time!

Cold Avocado Soup

Ingredients: 1 cucumber (approximately 1 lb.), 4 ripe avocados, 3 garlic cloves, 6 tablespoons heavy cream, ½ tablespoon flour, dash of lemon juice, 1 tablespoon cider vinegar, salt, pepper, 10 drops evening primrose oil, and 3 tablespoons crème fraîche.

Preparation: Peel the cucumber and the avocados, and cut them in half. Cut half of the cucumber and the avocados into small cubes. Place the other half, along with the garlic cloves, the heavy cream, the lemon juice, and the cider vinegar, into a blender, and purée. Season the soup with salt and pepper, and stir in the evening primrose oil. Divide the cucumber and the avocado cubes into two plates, and add the puréed mixture. Then garnish the soup with the crème fraîche.

Note: Avocados are rich in vitamin B6, which supports further processing of the gamma-linolenic acid in your body. This makes them an ideal supplement to a diet with evening primrose oil.

Fillets of Young Herring with a Sauce of Evening Primrose Oil and Sour Cream

Ingredients: 8 young herring fillets, 1 onion, 2 pickles, 2 apples, 1 tablespoon cider vinegar, 15 drops evening primrose oil, 12 oz. (350 g) sour cream, salt, pepper, and sugar or artificial sweetener.

Preparation: Cut the herring fillets into bite-size pieces and the onions into rings. Dice the pickles and the apples. Place all of the above ingredients into a bowl. Stir the cider vinegar along with the evening primrose oil in the sour cream, season to taste with salt, pepper, and sugar or artificial sweetener, and pour the sauce over the herring fillets. Allow them to marinate in the refrigerator for at least 2 hours before serving.

Fillets of young herring are rich in fatty acids contained in the fish oil and therefore augment the effect of evening primrose oil.

Asparagus Cocktail with Chicken

Ingredients: 10 oz. (300 g) chicken breast, 8 oz. (250 g) asparagus tips (from a can), 15 drops evening primrose oil, 5 tablespoons yogurt, 2 tablespoons hot mustard, 3 tablespoons lemon juice, 3.5 oz. (100 g) mayonnaise, salt, white pepper, cayenne, and dill.

Preparation: Boil the chicken breast, remove the skin, and cut the meat into small cubes. Place in cocktail glasses along with the drained asparagus tips. Stir the evening primrose oil into the yogurt, and mix with the mayonnaise together with the mustard and the lemon juice. Season the sauce with salt, white pepper, and cayenne, and pour over the asparagus tips and the chicken cubes. Garnish with finely chopped dill.

Zucchini with Tuna Filling

Ingredients: 4 zucchinis, 20 drops evening primrose oil, 3 tablespoons sour cream, 2 cans tuna (10.5 oz., or 300 g), 1 onion, 1½ tablespoons lemon juice, salt, and pepper.

Preparation: Blanch the zucchinis in boiling salted water; then refresh under cold running water. Cut in half, and remove the inner part of the zucchinis, reserving it. Stir the evening primrose oil into the sour cream, and place in blender along with the tuna, the chopped onion, the lemon juice, and the reserved zucchini pulp. Season with salt and pepper. Fill the paste into the hollowed-out zucchinis. Serve cold.

The Fitness Breakfast

Breakfast with Oats and Red Berries

Ingredients: 17.6 oz. (500 g) low-fat cottage cheese, 1 cup milk, 8 tablespoons rolled oats, 3 tablespoons red berries, 1 tablespoon grapes, 15 drops evening primrose oil, 2 tablespoons honey, and a little lemon juice.

Preparation: Stir the oats, the red berries, and the grapes into the low-fat cottage cheese and the milk, and add the evening primrose oil. Add the honey and the lemon juice to taste.

Rolled oats are rich in zinc, and lemon juice and red berries are an important source of vitamin C. The body needs both zinc and vitamin C in order to produce prostaglandin E1 from the dihomo-gamma-linolenic acid contained in evening primrose oil.

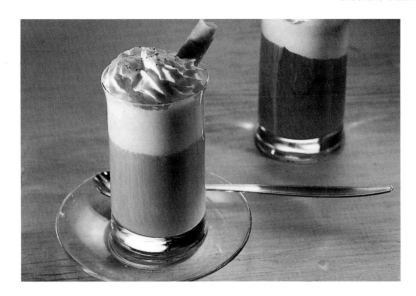

It's not just cold coffee—by adding evening primrose oil, you are doing something good for your health.

Delicious Desserts

Iced Coffee with Evening Primrose Oil and Whipped Cream

Ingredients: 1 cup heavy cream, 1 tablespoon sugar, 5 drops evening primrose oil, 4 scoops vanilla ice cream, 2 cups strong, refrigerated coffee, and 1 tablespoon instant-coffee powder.

Preparation: Whip the cream with the sugar, and then add the evening primrose oil. Fill four glasses (champagne glasses also work well) with 1 scoop each of the vanilla ice cream, and then add the coffee. Garnish with a dollop of the whipped cream, and sprinkle with the coffee powder.

Fruit Salad

Ingredients: 7 oz. (200 g) kiwi fruit, 7 oz. (200 g) peaches, 1 banana, 3.5 oz. (100 g) grapes, 3.5 oz. (100 g) pineapple pieces (from a can), sugar to taste, 1 cup heavy cream, and 5 drops evening primrose oil.

Preparation: Wash the fruit, peeling the kiwis and the peaches. Cut everything into bite-size pieces. Slice the peeled banana. Place all the fruit in a bowl. Sweeten to taste. Add the pineapple juice from the

Coffee is a good source of nicotine amide, which is required to convert dihomo-gamma-linolenic acid into prostaglandin E1. Coffee beans by themselves are already rich in nicotine amide. During roasting, the beans' content of nicotine amide is increased even further—one cup of coffee contains up to 2 milligrams of it.

can. Whip the cream, carefully stirring in the evening primrose oil, and pour this dressing over the fruit salad.

Note: The fruit contains a lot of vitamin C, which is important for the further processing of the evening primrose oil in the body. Cream is a natural emulsifier, ensuring that the evening primrose oil will blend evenly with the pineapple juice.

Orange Salad with Apples

Ingredients: 5 large oranges, 2 sweet apples, 4 tablespoons honey, 4 cloves, 1 cup water, 10 drops evening primrose oil, and 2 tablespoons vanilla sugar.

Preparation: Peel the oranges, removing all of the white skin parts. Cut in half and then into thin slices. Remove all seeds. Peel the apples, removing the cores. Cut them also into thin slices. Boil the honey with the cloves briefly in the water. Remove the cloves, and allow the honey mixture to simmer for several minutes more until it begins to thicken. Arrange the orange and apple slices in a circle on a plate, and glaze with the honey water. Sprinkle the vanilla sugar on top.

Note: Oranges and apples are rich in vitamin C, which is important to the body for the conversion of the essential fatty acids contained in evening primrose oil.

Lemon Cream

Ingredients: 1 unsprayed lemon, 3.5 oz. (100 g) sugar, 1 envelope unflavored gelatin, 1 cup heavy cream, and 10 drops evening primrose oil.

Preparation: Squeeze the juice out of the lemon (reserving the peel), and pour into a pan. Slightly heat the juice, stirring in the sugar. Grate half of the lemon peel, and add to the mixture in the pan. Dissolve the gelatin in 2 tablespoons of hot water, pass through a strainer, and add to the lemon juice. Whip the cream, add the evening primrose oil, and stir into the cooled-down lemon juice. Allow the cream to set in the refrigerator.

Note: This recipe contains a lot of vitamin C, which the body needs in order to convert the evening primrose oil.

Apples are a very valuable fruit: They stimulate the metabolism, activate the burning of fat, protect the blood vessels, detoxify the cells, and regulate the bowel functions.

Mango Cream with Pine Nuts and Evening Primrose Oil

Ingredients: 3 mangos, 2 eggs, 4 tablespoons sugar, 1½ tablespoons lemon juice, 1 envelope unflavored gelatin, 1 cup heavy cream, 15 drops evening primrose oil, and 3 tablespoons roasted pine nuts.

Preparation: Remove the fruit pulp from the mangos; dice a third of it, and purée the rest in a blender. Separate the eggs. Beat the egg yolks with the sugar until foamy, and stir into the puréed fruit along with the lemon juice. Dissolve the gelatin in a little water over a low heat, and add to the puréed fruit. Beat the egg whites until peaks will hold their shape, and add to the fruit mixture before it has set. Fill into dessert bowls, placing the mango cubes on top. Whip the cream until firm, stir in the evening primrose oil, and garnish the fruit with the cream. Sprinkle with the pine nuts.

Red Fruit Jelly with Evening Primrose Oil

Ingredients: 7 oz. (200 g) rhubarb, 7 oz. (200 g) currants, 7 oz. (200 g) gooseberries, 3.5 oz. (100 g) sugar, 1 cup water, 1.4 oz. (40 g) cornstarch, 1 cup heavy cream, and 15 drops evening primrose oil.

Preparation: Cook the rhubarb, the currants, and the gooseberries with the sugar and the water until they are soft and can be passed through a fine sieve. Add half of the cornstarch to the liquid pressed from the fruit. Bring this fruit mixture to a brief boil again, stirring in the other half of the cornstarch. Fill into four dessert bowls, and refrigerate. Whip the cream, stir in the evening primrose oil, and garnish the jelly with it prior to serving.

Mango, a subtropical fruit, is pleasantly sweet, juicy, and very refreshing.

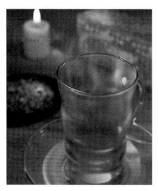

The tips of the stalks as well as the leaves from the evening primrose plant can be used to make a tea.

Evening primrose is often cultivated in English gardens. During the eighteenth century, not only was it a popular garden plant in Europe but it was also cultivated as a vegetable because of its tasty roots.

Additional Uses of the Evening Primrose Plant

More than just the oil from the evening primrose plant is good for our health. The Indians of North America and, for over a century now, also Western experts in natural healing methods have used different parts of the plant in the successful treatment of various ailments. In addition to the oil derived from its seeds, the tips of the stalks, the leaves, and the roots of the evening primrose plant can be used as a natural remedy and preventive.

Stalk Tips

The best time for harvesting the tips of the stalks is at the beginning of the blooming period, from June to July. Cut the blooming stalks about 4 to 8 inches (10 to 20 centimeters) below the blossoms. You can spread the tips in a well-ventilated place in your home and dry them by turning them daily. It's best to store the dried tips in small cloth sacks, in order to protect them from humidity.

Leaves

The leaves are harvested throughout the entire blooming period, from July through October. Dry the leaves in the open air, as per the instructions for drying the stalk tips. When the leaves are dry enough to be crumbled up between your fingers, break them up in this manner and store them also in small cloth sacks.

Boards of untreated wood that have been covered with linen cloth or blotting paper are especially suitable for the drying of the leaves and the tips. Frames made of wood and covered with a wire mesh also make an excellent drying surface.

Roots

Because evening primrose grows wild in many places, its tips and leaves are easy to gather and prepare. The roots should be dug up only when the seeds have formed in the fall or late fall, so that the plant can re-seed itself. Unlike the procedure for conserving the tips and the leaves, the roots from the evening primrose plant are not dried but can be used right away as a vegetable or a salad.

Healthful Recipes

Preparations with the Leaves and the Tips

A tea prepared from the leaves and the stalk tips of the evening primrose plant helps to alleviate various disorders, such as digestive problems, diarrhea, stomach and abdominal cramps, colds, and coughs. The tea also helps to generally enhance the liver function.

Tea

Ingredients: 1 tablespoon each of dried leaves and tips as well as 1 cup water.
Preparation: Pour the boiling water over the dried leaves and tips, and let the tea sit for 10 minutes. Stir occasionally, and then strain. You should drink two to three cups of this tea in small sips throughout the day and preferably without a sweetener.

Anti-inflammatory Topical Solution

Ingredients: 6 to 8 tablespoons dried leaves or tips (or a mixture of both) as well as 2 cups water.
Preparation: Add the evening primrose to the boiling water. Cover firmly with a lid, and let simmer over a low heat for 15 to 20 minutes. Strain the mixture carefully through a cloth or a sieve. Wash the affected parts of the body with this solution several times a day, and cover for 10 to 20 minutes with linen cloths that have been soaked in the solution.
Remember: This solution is meant for topical use only!

Because its flavor resembles that of ham, evening primrose was also known by the common name of ham root. The root, which grows up to 6 inches (15 centimeters) long, was cut into slices and served like ham. Prussian farmers during the eighteenth century used the evening primrose root as a flavorful vegetable or as a condiment or a salad.

Preparations with the Roots

According to an old legend, consuming 2 pounds of evening primrose roots will bring as much strength to the body as eating 20 pounds of beef. Whether or not that comparison is valid remains to be seen, but it is true that preparations from evening primrose roots do help to generally revitalize the body. They are especially suited to building up and strengthening the body after a lengthy illness or surgery. Due to the high protein, starch, and mineral content of the roots, a one- or two-week root cure in the fall is an excellent means to prepare for winter and to particularly stabilize the immune powers of the body.

So far there have been no reports of adverse effects caused by any parts of the evening primrose plant, regardless of whether evening primrose was used as a tea, in combination with other foods, or as a vegetable. Therefore, you may feel safe in using it to improve your health.

Basic Recipe for Root Vegetable and Root Salad

Ingredients: Approximately 1 lb. (500 g) scrubbed evening primrose roots, water, 1 tablespoon cider vinegar, salt, and pepper.
Preparation: Cut the roots into bite-size pieces. Place them in a pan, and add enough water to cover. Add the cider vinegar, and cook the roots until just firm. The roots can now be served with salt and pep-

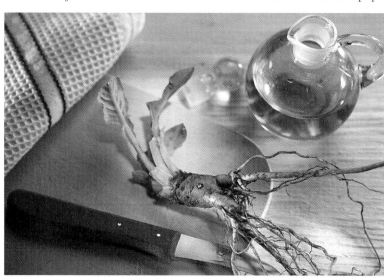

Evening primrose roots can enrich your menu, especially in wintertime or following an illness.

per, or they can be prepared in different ways as described in the following recipes.

Tip: This butter sauce is a tasty accompaniment to the roots:

Ingredients: 1 tablespoon butter, 1 tablespoon flour, ½ cup milk, and salt.

Preparation: Melt the butter, and stir in the flour. Thin with the milk, until the sauce reaches the desired consistency. Let simmer on a low heat for 10 minutes. You may add a small amount of cream if you wish.

Evening Primrose Root Salad with Chicken

Ingredients: To the basic recipe, add 7 oz. (200 g) frozen peas, 2 medium carrots sliced, pepper, 1 chicken breast (about ½ lb.), 1 bay leaf, 1 tablespoon hot mustard, salt, paprika, and 2 tablespoons thistle oil.

Preparation: Cook the peas with the carrots for approximately 8 minutes, drain, and mix with the roots. Boil the chicken breast, seasoned with pepper, and the bay leaf for 15 minutes on a low heat, and cut it into cubes. Stir the hot mustard into ½ cup of the cooking water from the roots, and season to taste with salt, pepper, and paprika. Add the thistle oil last. This marinade is then poured over the evening primrose roots, and it should be allowed to soak in for 30 minutes before the salad is served.

Tip: This salad is equally good served cold or warm. A fresh baguette goes particularly well with it.

Breaded Roots

Ingredients: To the basic recipe, add ½ cup milk, 1 egg, 1 tablespoon olive oil, 3.5 oz. (100 g) flour, salt, and oil for frying.

Preparation: Boil the roots, remove from the water, and dry them. Stir the milk, the egg, and the olive oil into the flour, and season with salt. The roots are then breaded with this mixture and fried in the hot oil until golden-yellow.

Roots au Gratin

Ingredients: To the basic recipe, add 5 oz. (150 g) sliced boiled ham, 1 tablespoon olive oil, and 3.5 oz. (100 g) Parmesan cheese.

The listed quantities are intended for two people.

Both evening primrose oil and thistle oil are rich in valuable linoleic acid. Because polyunsaturated fatty acids are very sensitive to heat, it is always best to use these high-grade oils uncooked whenever possible.

Preparation: Wrap the cooked evening primrose roots with the ham slices. Place the roots along with the olive oil into an ovenproof dish, and sprinkle with the Parmesan cheese. Bake the roots in a preheated oven at 400°F (200°C) until the cheese turns golden-brown.

Tip: In place of the Parmesan cheese, you may use pecorino, an Italian cheese made from goat's milk.

Evening Primrose Root Salad with Mushrooms and Watercress

Ingredients: To the basic recipe, add 1 garlic clove, 2 shallots, 2 tablespoons wine vinegar, 3 tablespoons olive oil, salt, pepper, 8 oz. (250 g) small whole or large quartered mushrooms, and 1 bunch watercress.

Preparation: Finely mince the garlic and the shallots. Prepare a marinade from the wine vinegar and the olive oil, adding the garlic and the shallots. Season to taste with salt and pepper. Now add the mushrooms to the evening primrose roots. Trim and wash the watercress, and add to the mushrooms and the roots. Pour the marinade over the salad, and toss.

Tip: This root salad is especially good accompanied by a fresh baguette or a ciabatta, an Italian type of white bread with a hard crust and a fluffy dough.

Some people are turned off by its odor, but garlic has proven to be excellent for our health. Its benefits for the cardiovascular system and in bacterial or viral infections are undisputed.